Nursing Skills in Control and Coordination

T0091630

Looking at how a variety of biological systems control and coordinate all physical actions, this quick reference book covers the nervous system and neurological assessment, caring for the unconscious patient and dealing with pain. Suitable for student nurses and nursing associates, it is ideal for use in practice. This practical pocket guide covers:

- the anatomy and physiology of the nervous system
- neurological assessment
- caring for the unconscious patient
- pain assessment and management
- sleep.

This competency-based text covers relevant key concepts, anatomy and physiology, lifespan matters, assessment and nursing skills. To support your learning, it also includes learning outcomes, concept map summaries, activities, questions and scenarios with sample answers and critical reflection thinking points.

Quick and easy to reference, this short, clinically-focused guide is ideal for use on placements or for revision. It is suitable for pre-registration nurses, students on the nursing associate programme and newly qualified nurses.

Tina Moore is a Senior Lecturer in Adult Nursing at Middlesex University, UK. She teaches nursing assessment, clinical skills and care interventions for both pre-qualifying and post-qualifying nurses. She is also a Middlesex University Teaching Fellow.

Sheila Cunningham is an Associate Professor in Adult Nursing at Middlesex University, UK. She has a breadth of experience teaching nurses both pre- and post-registration and she mentors clinicians supporting students in practice. She is also a Middlesex University Teaching Fellow and holds a Principal Fellowship at the Higher Education Academy. Her current role is Director for Learning, Teaching and Quality (School of Health and Education).

Skills in Nursing Practice

Series editors
Tina Moore, *Middlesex University, UK*
Sheila Cunningham, *Middlesex University, UK*

This series of competency-based pocket guides covers relevant key concepts, anatomy and physiology, lifespan matters, assessment and nursing skills for good clinical practice in a range of areas from safety and protection to promoting homeostasis. To support your learning, they include learning outcomes, concept map summaries, activities, questions and scenarios with sample answers and critical reflection thinking points.

Quick and easy to reference, these short, skills-focused texts are ideal for use on placements or for revision. They are ideal for pre-registration nurses, students on the nursing associate programme and newly qualified nurses feeling in need of a little revision.

List of Titles:

Nursing Skills in Professional and Practice Contexts
Tina Moore and Sheila Cunningham

Nursing Skills in Safety and Protection
Sheila Cunningham and Tina Moore

Nursing Skills in Nutrition, Hydration and Elimination
Sheila Cunningham and Tina Moore

Nursing Skills in Cardiorespiratory Assessment and Monitoring
Tina Moore and Sheila Cunningham

Nursing Skills in Supporting Mobility
Sheila Cunningham and Tina Moore

Nursing Skills in Control and Coordination
Tina Moore and Sheila Cunningham

For more information about this series, please visit: www.routle dge.com/Skills-in-Nursing-Practice/book-series/SNP

Nursing Skills in Control and Coordination

**Tina Moore and
Sheila Cunningham**

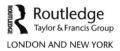
Routledge
Taylor & Francis Group

LONDON AND NEW YORK

First published 2021
by Routledge
2 Park Square, Milton Park, Abingdon, Oxon OX14 4RN

and by Routledge
605 Third Avenue, New York, NY 10158

Routledge is an imprint of the Taylor & Francis Group, an informa business

British Library Cataloguing-in-Publication Data
A catalogue record for this book is available from the British Library

Library of Congress Cataloging-in-Publication Data
Names: Moore, Tina, 1962- author. | Cunningham, Sheila, author.
Title: Nursing skills in control and coordination / Tina Moore, Sheila
Cunningham.
Description: New York: Routledge, 2021. | Series: Skills in nursing
practice | Includes bibliographical references and index. |
Summary: "Looking at how a variety of biological systems control and
coordinate all physical actions, this quick reference book covers the nervous
system and neurological assessment, caring for the unconscious patient
and dealing with pain. Suitable for student nurses and nursing
associates, it is ideal for use in practice. Quick and easy to
reference, this short, clinically-focused guide is ideal for use on
placements or for revision. It is suitable for pre-registration nurses,
students on the nursing associate programme and newly qualified
nurses"– Provided by publisher.
Identifiers: LCCN 2020047460 (print) | LCCN 2020047461 (ebook) |
ISBN 9781138479364 (hardback) | ISBN 9781138479371 (paperback) |
ISBN 9781351065900 (ebook)
Subjects: LCSH: Neurological nursing. | Nursing assessment.
Classification: LCC RC350.5 .M66 2021 (print) | LCC RC350.5 (ebook) |
DDC 616.8/04231–dc23
LC record available at https://lccn.loc.gov/2020047460
LC ebook record available at https://lccn.loc.gov/2020047461

ISBN: 978-1-138-47936-4 (hbk)
ISBN: 978-1-138-47937-1 (pbk)
ISBN: 978-1-351-06590-0 (ebk)

Typeset in Stone Serif
By Deanta Global Publishing Services, Chennai, India

Contents

Figures

FIGURES

Introduction to the *Skills in Nursing Practice* series

This particular book is one in a series of six *'Nursing Skills in...'* books.

Book 1 *Professional Skills and Practice Context*
Book 2 *Protection and Safety*
Book 3 *Acquisition of Nutrients and Removal of Waste*
Book 4 *Control and Co-ordination*
Book 5 *Cardiorespiratory Assessment and Monitoring*
Book 6 *Supporting Mobility*

These books are designed to be used in clinical practice and can be used not only for reference but also as an invaluable revision tool. There is a continuing emphasis on skills acquisition and development particularly within nursing. This is accompanied by the increasing understanding of the necessity to effectively and efficiently integrate theory and clinical skill competence-based learning. In doing so, these books hope to ensure that nurses have the best opportunity to become fit to practice and develop key employability skills. Therefore, each chapter has been linked to the *Future Nurse Proficiencies* (NMC 2018) which will enable you to map your skills development in relation to the standards set by the professional body.

The structure of each chapter within the books draws on constructivist pedagogical approaches and assimilation theory. Each chapter presents interlinking ideas and information through the use of concept maps. It is anticipated that the use of key words and connections will deepen and enhance those linkages from the concepts, drawing on the general and specific aspects of a topic, and will therefore promote active learning.

Concept maps are pictures or graphic representations that will help you to organise and represent your knowledge of a subject. This is achieved through helping you to link, differentiate and relate concepts to one another. They (concept maps) begin with a main idea (or concept) and then branch out to show how that main idea can be broken down into specific topics. They can also visually represent relationships between concepts and ideas in a quick, easy-to-understand format. Concept mapping is becoming increasingly popular as a means of teaching and learning within education. The introduction of concept maps will provide a quick summary with additional key information about the material in the *Clinical Skills for Nursing* book. We have also included related anatomy and physiology together with lifespan matters.

The end of each chapter will have questions (answers also provided) in the format of a quiz. This will help you to test your new knowledge, understanding and application of the content. There is also the opportunity for you to critically reflect on your learning using the SMART (Specific, Measurable, Achievable, Realistic and Time-bound) format. From this you should then be able to clearly identify areas for future development and learning.

These pocket-size books are not only designed to help develop your clinical skills (practice and knowledge) but also to improve your key transferrable skills, enabling them to advance your employability skills, i.e. problem solving; analytical and critical thinking; and team working. Therefore another aim for each book is to concentrate on scaffolding learning, therefore supporting, promoting and developing autonomous learning, questioning (informed) and critical thinking. The use of concept mapping allows the reorganisation of information in a visual manner to promote critical thinking in the nursing student. Through concept mapping students can see how ideas and patient care needs, and the interrelationships that exist between them, promote critical thinking in relation to clinical practice.

The books within this series are not designed to be comprehensive textbooks. They are the practice companions of the *Clinical Skills for Nursing Practice*, and are designed to be used in conjunction with that book. The design of these 'pocket-size' books will enable students/readers to use them as a resource whilst working within and outside of clinical practice.

Tina Moore and Sheila Cunningham

Introduction and overview

The body needs to coordinate effectively and efficiently in order to function as a whole, that is, all the systems of the body working together to maintain homeostasis and function. Through controlled coordination between stimuli and the body's responses and adapting to change, the body can avoid injury and danger.

For survival, the human body has to adjust to its surrounding external and internal environments and stimuli. A living being does not live in isolation. It has to constantly interact with its external environment and has to respond properly for its survival.

In order for these adjustments to be made, it is essential that the mechanism of control and coordination involve many systems of the human body working together synchronously. There are two types of coordination, nervous (controlled by the nervous system) and hormonal (controlled by the endocrine system).

Collectively, the nervous and endocrine systems work harmoniously and together are responsible for the control and coordination of complex, multicellular, multiple organ systems. Jointly, they control and coordinate all physical actions, homeostasis, thinking processes and emotional behaviours.

The nervous system permits the continuing performance in daily activities by facilitating the response to the body's environment. This is achieved by the transmission of sensory information to the central nervous system from external and internal stimuli. This in turn influences involuntary and voluntary (motor) actions. Likewise, hormones are secreted from the endocrine system and regulate the growth, development and functioning of different organs.

When these processes are compromised, the body becomes challenged and may progress into a state of illness, injury or

3

disability. Whilst there are many patient problems that fall into these categories (too many for the purpose of this book) only the most common areas that are likely to be experienced by student nurses will be discussed. These include alterations to the level of consciousness, assessment of level of consciousness, caring for the unconscious patient, pain and sleep. This book should be read in conjunction with *Clinical Skills for Nursing Practice*.

CHAPTER 1

Overview of the nervous system functions

Sheila Cunningham

Overview

The control and coordination of the human body depends on many interacting systems and tissues. The key one is the nervous system which detects and responds to changes inside and outside the body. Together with the endocrine system, it monitors and regulates vital aspects of body functions and maintains homeostasis. Stable internal environments are important in health and disruption can be challenging and requires expert nursing and medical attention. The nervous system is also associated with higher order functions such as learning, thinking, decision-making and consciousness. It is therefore necessary to look at the fundamental structures and processes to explore how these develop and how we (including patients) make sense of the world.

Link to *Future Nurse Proficiencies* (NMC 2018)

Annexe A: Section 2: Procedures for the planning, provision and management of person-centred nursing care. Specifically, 2.1: share information and check understanding about the causes, implications and treatment of a range of common health conditions including anxiety, depression, memory loss, diabetes, dementia, respiratory disease, cardiac disease, neurological disease, cancer, skin problems, immune efficiencies, psychosis, stroke and arthritis.

Annexe B, Part 1: Specifically, 2.7: undertake a whole body systems assessment including respiratory, circulatory, neurological, musculoskeletal, cardiovascular and skin status and 2.12: undertake, respond to and interpret neurological observations and assessments.

Expected knowledge

- Terminology related to communicating the nervous system functions
- Fundamental differences between the central and peripheral nervous system
- Role of the nervous system in maintenance of homeostasis.

Introduction

Homeostasis is vital to human functioning as well as wellbeing and health. It is maintained through the coordinated actions of the nervous and endocrine systems in a dynamic and unceasing manner. As well as monitoring and responding to changes in the internal and external environment, the nervous system is also responsible for sensory perception, behaviour, memory and involuntary and voluntary movements. As such there are very few areas within nursing and health care where aspects of nervous functioning are not relevant. Developmental changes occur throughout the lifespan and thus the functioning is not static and improvements as well as deteriorations occur which the nurse ought to be aware of to support or care for people undergoing such changes. Fundamentally, it requires a depth of knowledge, not just of applications but also of the key structures and functions of the nervous system, to ensure a comprehensive knowledge and evidence base to inform decisions on care approaches.

The health care needs of patients within the hospital setting and the community are becoming increasingly complex. Several activities of daily living involve aspects of nervous functioning: sleep, breathing, elimination, movement, feeling safe and secure. Each has a sequence of actions and mechanisms to it and knowing the normal and detecting the abnormal are imperative to ensuring and maintaining these activities. Modern living is such that people are living longer with neurological issues and the capacity of the nervous system to adapt and readjust is immense; however, it has limits. This requires health care professionals including nurses to have the appropriate knowledge and skill in order to manage any neurological changes and deficits, and to understand normal neurological functioning and development as well as how to test for and interpret neurological or sensory functioning.

Content

Structural and functional divisions of the nervous system	Central control of nervous functions	Somatosensory developments and mapping
Higher order functions: memory, thoughts and learning	Nerve communication: action potentials and synapses	Neurotransmitters and application to nursing

Learning outcomes

- Outline and describe the structure of the nervous system and component parts
- Differentiate higher order versus lower order functioning of the nervous system
- Briefly explain changes in nervous system development throughout the life span
- Explain what is meant by the somatosensory nervous system and how nurses might evaluate its functioning
- Describe and appraise the role of learning and emotional development
- Reflect on your knowledge on nervous system physiology, pathology and pharmacology and ways to enhance it.

Key background

The range of people with neurological issues is vast and their issues vary from physical to processing or emotional. There is a branch of nursing, 'Neuroscience nursing', which focuses on caring for people with a variety of neurological conditions and disorders across the lifespan and in all health care settings. This is a specialist area of nursing (see RCN, 2020 Neuroscience network), though the ranges of patients and care environments are familiar to many nurses: neurological surgery or neurological trauma, for example brain and spinal cord injury; critical/intensive care; long-term neurological conditions, such as stroke (cerebrovascular accident), multiple sclerosis, Parkinson's Disease, or epilepsy; or life-restricting conditions, such as motor neurone disease. People with these conditions may live long lives and be in the community, care home or hospital settings. There are also mental health nurses who deal with the consequences of neurological problems and processing or affective issues, all of which point to a fundamental need to have a firm grasp of the nervous system functions. As with many conditions these are not necessarily static and understanding the mechanism of development or deterioration is key. Later chapters in this book address issues of consciousness, coma or perception of pain or sleep. These are applications and the first chapter addresses the overview of the structures and processes to set the later chapters in context. Anatomy and physiology can be perceived as very 'dry' areas; however, nurses and health care professionals have the advantage of seeing it 'live' in our patients and work environments and also within our own family environments. Thinking and sensations are fundamental to all of us and so is included in here to enable application of and excitement about this tricky topic.

NERVOUS SYSTEM REVIEW AND OVERVIEW

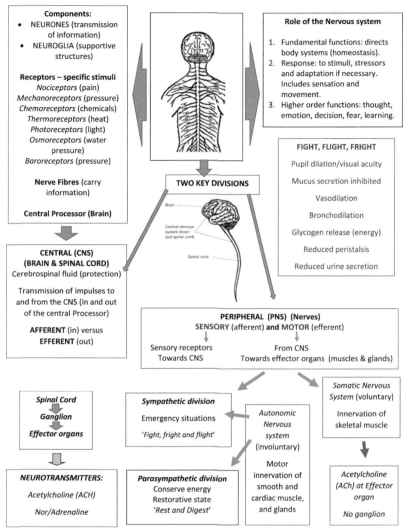

Components:
- NEURONES (transmission of information)
- NEUROGLIA (supportive structures)

Receptors – specific stimuli
Nociceptors (pain)
Mechanoreceptors (pressure)
Chemoreceptors (chemicals)
Thermoreceptors (heat)
Photoreceptors (light)
Osmoreceptors (water pressure)
Baroreceptors (pressure)

Nerve Fibres (carry information)

Central Processor (Brain)

Role of the Nervous system

1. Fundamental functions: directs body systems (homeostasis).
2. Response: to stimuli, stressors and adaptation if necessary. Includes sensation and movement.
3. Higher order functions: thought, emotion, decision, fear, learning.

TWO KEY DIVISIONS

FIGHT, FLIGHT, FRIGHT

Pupil dilation/visual acuity

Mucus secretion inhibited

Vasodilation

Bronchodilation

Glycogen release (energy)

Reduced peristalsis

Reduced urine secretion

CENTRAL (CNS)
(BRAIN & SPINAL CORD)
Cerebrospinal fluid (protection)

Transmission of impulses to and from the CNS (in and out of the central Processor)

AFFERENT (in) versus
EFFERENT (out)

PERIPHERAL (PNS) (Nerves)
SENSORY (afferent) **and** MOTOR (efferent)

Sensory receptors
Towards CNS

From CNS
Towards effector organs (muscles & glands)

Spinal Cord
↓
Ganglion
↓
Effector organs

Sympathetic division

Emergency situations

'Fight, fright and flight'

Autonomic Nervous system (involuntary)

Motor innervation of smooth and cardiac muscle, and glands

Somatic Nervous System (voluntary)

Innervation of skeletal muscle

NEUROTRANSMITTERS:

Acetylcholine (ACH)

Nor/Adrenaline

Parasympathetic division
Conserve energy
Restorative state
'Rest and Digest'

Acetylcholine (ACh) at Effector organ

No ganglion

FIGURE 1.1 Overview and review of the nervous system

NEUROTRANSMISSION

Also termed *Action Potential*

- The conduction of nerve impulses.
- Occurs through detection of stimuli in the form of electrochemical impulses.
- Electrical transmission occurs along the nerve fibre.
- Each neuron has electrical potential resulting from separation of ions: Sodium (Na+) inside the cell and Potassium (K+) outside the cell.

At rest = POLARISED OR

INSIDE = Positively charged

OUTSIDE = Negatively charged

- Stimulation alters membrane permeability to Na+, it enters the cell causing **DEPOLARISATION**.

INSIDE = Negatively charged

OUTSIDE = Positively charged

- Impulse spread is increased permeability along the fibre until normality restored) **ACTION POTENTIAL**

- At axon end **CHEMICAL** transmission (**Neurotransmitters**) occurs (**SYNAPSE**) to adjoining nerve or muscle then chemical is broken down or reabsorbed to prevent sustained transmission.

- **Sensory** impulses – BRAIN (interpretation)
- **Motor** Impulse – muscle/organ (action)
- Speed of transmission due to axon diameter, length and myelin

Fibre Categories:

- *A fibre = fastest (e.g. touch).*
- *C fibre = slowest (e.g. pain).*

NERVE IMPULSES AND SENSES

NEURONE

Three distinct areas: *Dendrites* (receiving), *Soma* (body) and *Axon* (transmitting fibre):

IMPULSE DIRECTION

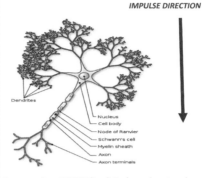

Axon covering = **MYELIN** (insulation) speeds up impulse transmission

Nicolas.Rougier / CC BY-SA (http://creativecommons.org/licenses/by-sa/3.0/)

SENSORY SYSTEMS

Sensation is a *'state of awareness of external and internal conditions of the body'* (Tortora & Derrickson 2019 p. 276)

Three conditions must be present:
1. Stimulus
2. Receptor or sense organ
3. Impulse conducted

A region of the brain to interpret/translate the sensation. Receptors convert specific stimulus (e.g. light, chemical energy or pressure) and convert it to a nerve impulse. Receptors may be simple (fibres) or complex (bulb structures).

Direction to the brain is via an afferent pathway in the spinal cord to a sensory area in the cerebral cortex.

Sensory characteristics:
- Projection (locates) sensation
- Adaptation (decrease sensitivity)
- 'After images' (sensation persists after stimulus removed)
- Modality (specificity to type of sensation transmitted).

Two main types of sensory systems

General: receptors are found widely in the body
Special: receptors are found in complex organs in small body

FIGURE 1.2 Nerve impulses and senses

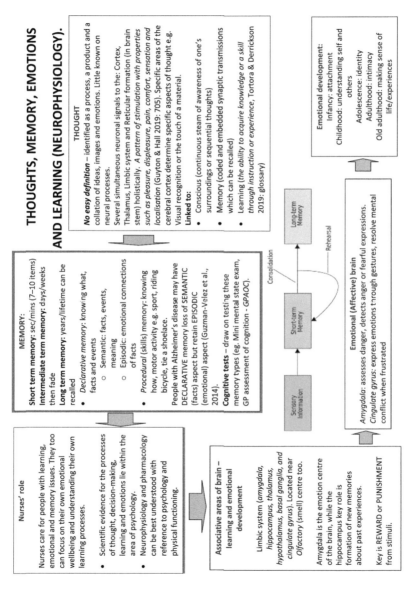
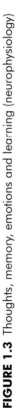

THOUGHTS, MEMORY, EMOTIONS AND LEARNING (NEUROPHYSIOLOGY).

THOUGHT

No easy definition – identified as a process, a product and a collation of ideas, images and emotions. Little known on neural processes.

Several simultaneous neuronal signals to the: Cortex, Thalamus, Limbic system and Reticular formation (in brain stem) holistically. *A pattern of stimulation with properties such as pleasure, displeasure, pain, comfort, sensation and localisation* (Guyton & Hall 2019: 705). Specific areas of the cerebral cortex determine specific aspects of thought e.g. Visual recognition or the touch of a material.

Linked to:

- Conscious (continuous steam of awareness of one's surroundings or sequential thoughts)
- Memory (coded and embedded synaptic transmissions which can be recalled)
- Learning (*the ability to acquire knowledge or a skill through instruction or experience*, Tortora & Derrickson 2019: glossary)

Nurses' role

Nurses care for people with learning, emotional and memory issues. They too can focus on their own emotional wellbeing and understanding their own learning processes.

- Scientific evidence for the processes of thought, decision-making, learning and emotions lie within the area of psychology.
- Neurophysiology and pharmacology can be best understood with reference to psychology and physical functioning.

MEMORY:

Short term memory: sec/mins (7–10 items)
Intermediate term memory: days/weeks then fade
Long term memory: years/lifetime can be recalled

- *Declarative memory:* knowing what, facts and events
  - Semantic: facts, events, meaning
  - Episodic: emotional connections of facts
- *Procedural* (skills) memory: knowing how, motor activity e.g. sport, riding bicycle, tie a shoelace.

People with Alzheimer's disease may have DECLARATIVE memory loss of SEMANTIC (facts) aspect but retain EPISODIC (emotional) aspect (Guzman-Velez et al., 2014).

Cognitive tests – draw on testing these memory types (eg. Mini mental state exam, GP assessment of cognition - GPAOC).

Associative areas of brain – learning and emotional development

Limbic system (*amygdala, hippocampus, thalamus, hypothalamus, basal ganglia, and cingulate gyrus*). Located near *Olfactory* (smell) centre too.

Amygdala is the emotion centre of the brain, while the hippocampus key role is formation of new memories about past experiences.

Key is REWARD or PUNISHMENT from stimuli.

Emotional (Affective) brain

Amygdala: assesses danger, detects anger or fearful expressions.
Cingulate gyrus: express emotions through gestures, resolve mental conflict when frustrated

Emotional development:

Infancy: attachment
Childhood: understanding self and others
Adolescence: identity
Adulthood: intimacy
Old adulthood: making sense of life/experiences

Sensory Information → Short-term Memory → Long-term Memory
Consolidation
Rehearsal

FIGURE 1.3 Thoughts, memory, emotions and learning (neurophysiology)

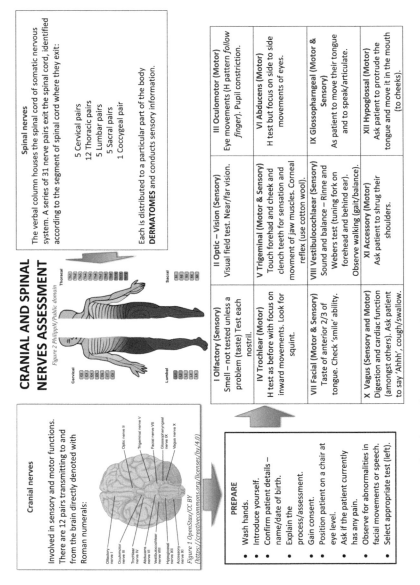

Cranial nerves

Involved in sensory and motor functions. There are 12 pairs transmitting to and from the brain directly denoted with Roman numerals:

Figure 1 OpenStax/CC BY (https://creativecommons.org/licenses/by/4.0)

CRANIAL AND SPINAL NERVES ASSESSMENT

Figure 2 PhilipN/Public domain

Spinal nerves

The verbal column houses the spinal cord of somatic nervous system. A series of 31 nerve pairs exit the spinal cord, identified according to the segment of spinal cord where they exit:

- 5 Cervical pairs
- 12 Thoracic pairs
- 5 Lumbar pairs
- 5 Sacral pairs
- 1 Coccygeal pair

Each is distributed to a particular part of the body DERMATOMES and conducts sensory information.

PREPARE

- Wash hands.
- Introduce yourself.
- Confirm patient details – name/date of birth.
- Explain the process/assessment.
- Gain consent.
- Position patient on a chair at eye level.
- Ask if the patient currently has any pain.
- Observe for abnormalities in facial movements or speech.
- Select appropriate test (left).

I Olfactory (Sensory)	II Optic – Vision (Sensory)	III Oculomotor (Motor)
Smell – not tested unless a problem (taste) Test each nostril.	Visual field test. Near/far vision.	Eye movements (H pattern follow finger). Pupil constriction.
IV Trochlear (Motor)	V Trigeminal (Motor & Sensory)	VI Abducens (Motor)
H test as before with focus on inward movements. Look for squint.	Touch forehad and cheek and clench teeth for sensation and movment of jaw muscles. Corneal reflex (use cotton wool).	H test but focus on side to side movements of eyes.
VII Facial (Motor & Sensory)	VIII Vestibulocochlaear (Sensory)	IX Glossopharngeal (Motor & Sensory)
Taste of anterior 2/3 of tongue. Check 'smile' ability.	Sound and balance – Rinne and Webers test (tuning fork on forehead and behind ear). Observe walking (gait/balance).	As patient to move their tongue and to speak/articulate.
X Vagus (Sensory and Motor)	XI Accessory (Motor)	XII Hypoglossal (Motor)
Digestion and cardiac function (amongst others). Ask patient to say 'Ahhh', cough/swallow.	Ask patient to shrug their shoulders.	Ask patient to protrude the tongue and move it in the mouth (to cheeks).

FIGURE 1.4 Cranial and spinal nerve assessment

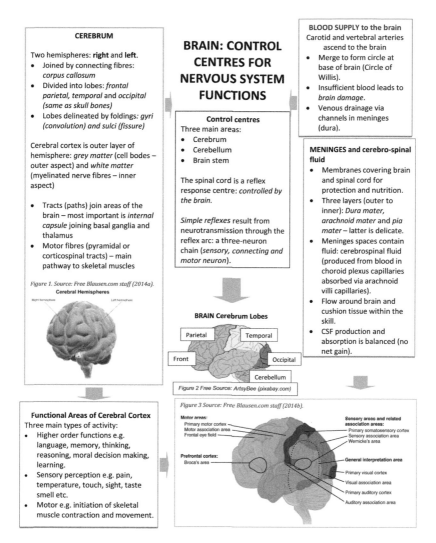

CEREBRUM

Two hemispheres: **right** and **left**.
- Joined by connecting fibres: *corpus callosum*
- Divided into lobes: *frontal parietal, temporal* and *occipital (same as skull bones)*
- Lobes delineated by foldings: *gyri (convolution) and sulci (fissure)*

Cerebral cortex is outer layer of hemisphere: *grey matter* (cell bodes – outer aspect) and *white matter* (myelinated nerve fibres – inner aspect)

- Tracts (paths) join areas of the brain – most important is *internal capsule* joining basal ganglia and thalamus
- Motor fibres (pyramidal or corticospinal tracts) – main pathway to skeletal muscles

Figure 1. Source: Free Blausen.com staff (2014a).
Cerebral Hemispheres

BRAIN: CONTROL CENTRES FOR NERVOUS SYSTEM FUNCTIONS

Control centres
Three main areas:
- Cerebrum
- Cerebellum
- Brain stem

The spinal cord is a reflex response centre: *controlled by the brain.*

Simple reflexes result from neurotransmission through the reflex arc: a three-neuron chain (*sensory, connecting and motor neuron*).

BRAIN Cerebrum Lobes

Parietal   Temporal

Front   Occipital

Cerebellum

Figure 2 Free Source: ArtsyBee (pixabay.com)

BLOOD SUPPLY to the brain
Carotid and vertebral arteries ascend to the brain
- Merge to form circle at base of brain (Circle of Willis).
- Insufficient blood leads to *brain damage.*
- Venous drainage via channels in meninges (dura).

MENINGES and cerebro-spinal fluid
- Membranes covering brain and spinal cord for protection and nutrition.
- Three layers (outer to inner): *Dura mater, arachnoid mater* and *pia mater* – latter is delicate.
- Meninges spaces contain fluid: cerebrospinal fluid (produced from blood in choroid plexus capillaries absorbed via arachnoid villi capillaries).
- Flow around brain and cushion tissue within the skill.
- CSF production and absorption is balanced (no net gain).

Functional Areas of Cerebral Cortex
Three main types of activity:
- Higher order functions e.g. language, memory, thinking, reasoning, moral decision making, learning.
- Sensory perception e.g. pain, temperature, touch, sight, taste smell etc.
- Motor e.g. initiation of skeletal muscle contraction and movement.

Figure 3 Source: Free Blausen.com staff (2014b).

Motor areas:
Primary motor cortex
Motor association area
Frontal eye field

Prefrontal cortex:
Broca's area

Sensory areas and related association areas:
Primary somatosensory cortex
Sensory association area
Wernicke's area

General interpretation area

Primary visual cortex
Visual association area
Primary auditory cortex
Auditory association area

FIGURE 1.5 Brain: control centres for nervous system functions

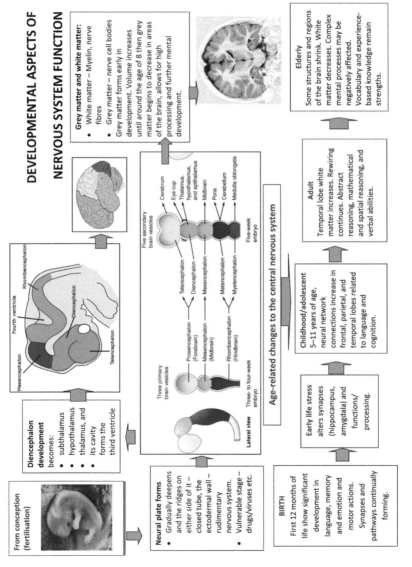

DEVELOPMENTAL ASPECTS OF NERVOUS SYSTEM FUNCTION

From conception (fertilisation)

Neural plate forms
- Gradually deepens and the ridges on either side of it – closed tube, the ectodermal wall – rudimentary nervous system.
- Vulnerable stage – drugs/viruses etc.

Diencephalon development becomes:
- subthalamus
- hypothalamus
- thalamus, and its cavity – forms the third ventricle

Mesencephalon
Fourth ventricle
Rhombencephalon
Diencephalon
Telencephalon

Grey matter and white matter:
- White matter – Myelin, nerve fibres
- Grey matter – nerve cell bodies

Grey matter forms early in development. Volume increases until around the age of 8 then grey matter begins to decrease in areas of the brain, allows for high processing and further mental development.

Three primary brain vesicles

Prosencephalon (Forebrain) → Telencephalon
Diencephalon
Mesencephalon (Midbrain) → Mesencephalon
Rhombencephalon (Hindbrain) → Metencephalon
Myelencephalon

Lateral view
Three- to four-week embryo

Five secondary brain vesicles

Cerebrum
Eye cup
Thalamus, hypothalamus, and epithalamus
Midbrain
Pons
Cerebellum
Medulla oblongata

Five-week embryo

Age-related changes to the central nervous system

BIRTH
First 12 months of life show significant development in language, memory and emotion and motor actions. Synapses and pathways continually forming.

Early life stress alters synapses (hippocampus, amygdala) and functions/processing.

Childhood/adolescent
5–11 years of age, neural network connections increase in frontal, parietal, and temporal lobes related to language and cognition.

Adult
Temporal lobe white matter increases. Rewiring continues. Abstract reasoning, mathematical and spatial reasoning, and verbal abilities.

Elderly
Some structures and regions of the brain shrink. White matter decreases. Complex mental processes may be negatively affected. Vocabulary and experience-based knowledge remain strengths.

FIGURE 1.6 Developmental aspects of nervous system function

NEUROTRANSMITTERS: NURSING IMPLICATIONS

Types and actions of NTs

Several (>50) of which 10 are important:

- *Acetylcholine* (ACh)
- Monoamines: *norepinephrine (NE), dopamine (DA), serotonin (5-HT)*, melatonin
- Amino acids: *glutamate, gamma aminobutyric acid (GABA), aspartate, glycine, histamine*
- Purines: *Adenosine, ATP, GTP*, and their derivatives

They can be:

- **EXCITATORY** – stimulate (fight and flight, motor, stimulate thinking etc. Too much causes restlessness, anxiety etc.) e.g. Dopamine, Histamine, Norepinephrine, Epinephrine
- **INHIBITORY** – decrease excitation (induce sleep, calm, rest) e.g. GABA, Dopamine, Serotonin

Acetylcholine

First neurotransmitter discovered – found in the brain, spinal cord and particularly at the neuromuscular junction of the skeletal muscle.

- Can act excitatory or inhibitory.
- Synthesized from dietary choline (red meat and vegetables).

Alzheimer's disease linked with decreased ACh in neurons.

Physiologic effects and functions:

- Muscular stimulation – acetylcholine signals muscles to become active.
- Controls the sleep and wakefulness cycle – scheduling the rapid eye movement (REM) sleep or dream.

Neurotransmitters (NT) are chemicals released during a synapse to initiate an impulse on the adjacent Neuron or Muscle/Organ.

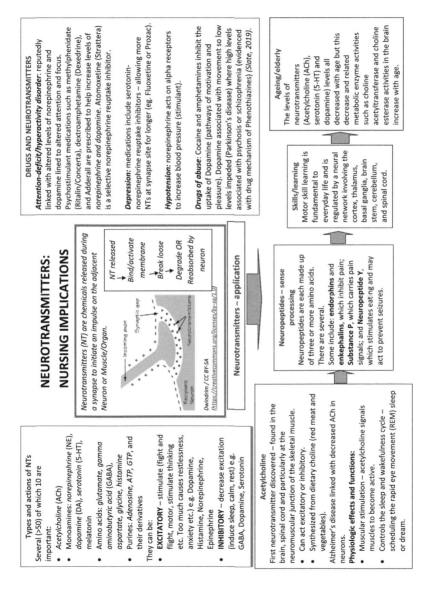

Dwindrin / CC BY-SA
(https://creativecommons.org/licenses/by-sa/1.0)

NT released
Bind/activate membrane
Break loose
Degrade OR
Reabsorbed by neuron

Neurotransmitters – application

Neuropeptides – sense processing

Neuropeptides are each made up of three or more amino acids. There are several. Some include: **endorphins** and **enkephalins**, which inhibit pain; **Substance P**, which carries pain signals; and **Neuropeptide Y**, which stimulates eating and may act to prevent seizures.

Skills/learning

Motor skill learning is fundamental to everyday life and is regulated by a neural network involving the cortex, thalamus, basal ganglia, brain stem, cerebellum, and spinal cord.

DRUGS AND NEUROTRANSMITTERS

Attention-deficit/hyperactivity disorder: reputedly linked with altered levels of norepinephrine and dopamine linked to altered attention and focus. Psychostimulant medications such as methylphenidate (Ritalin/Concerta), dextroamphetamine (Dexedrine), and Adderall are prescribed to help increase levels of *norepinephrine and dopamine.* Atomoxetine (Strattera) is a selective norepinephrine reuptake inhibitor.

Depression: medications include serotonin-norepinephrine reuptake inhibitors – allowing more NTs at synapse site for longer (eg. Fluoxetine or Prozac).

Hypotension: norepinephrine acts on alpha receptors to increase blood pressure (stimulant).

Drugs of abuse: Cocaine and amphetamines inhibit the uptake of Dopamine (pathways of motivation and pleasure). Dopamine associated with movement so low levels of Dopamine impeded (Parkinson's disease) where high levels associated with psychosis or schizophrenia (evidenced with drug mechanism of Phenothiazines) *(Slate, 2019).*

Ageing/elderly

The levels of neurotransmitters (Acetylcholine (ACh), serotonin (5-HT) and dopamine) levels all decreased with age but this decrease and related metabolic enzyme activities such as choline acetyltransferase and choline esterase activities in the brain increase with age.

FIGURE 1.7 Neurotransmitters

Activity: now test yourself

1. The autonomic nervous system refers to one part of the nervous system structure. Which of the following is it?

   a) part of the brain and regulatory structures

   b) a component of the peripheral nervous system responsible for voluntary movement

   c) part of the spinal cord that links the central and peripheral nervous system nerves together

   d) developed in later life in response to nervous system maturity

   e) part of the peripheral nervous system responsible for involuntary controls such as thermoregulation or vasoconstriction.

2. Identify which of the following statements is **true** or **false**.

Statement	True or false
Afferent nerves carry impulses towards the central nervous system.	
Skeletal muscles are the only effector organs of the somatic nervous system.	
The dura mater is the fine innermost layer of the meninges that completely covers the brain.	
The vestibulocochlear nerves are associated with hearing, posture and balance.	

3. The special senses do not include which of the following?

   a) pain

   b) balance

   c) sight

   d) taste.

4. Match the letter in List A with the number description in List B.

	List A	Answer
a)	cerebral cortex	
b)	corpus callosum	
c)	dermatome	
d)	white matter	
e)	myelin	

	List B
1	mass of white matter that connects the two cerebral hemispheres
2	superficial part of the cerebrum
3	formed by bodies of nerve cells (not fibres)
4	produced by Schwann cells and forming an outer layer of axons to aid conduction and insulation of impulses
5	area of skin whose sensory receptors are associated with a specific nerve

5. Neurotransmitters are nerve chemicals involved in synaptic transmission (propagation of impulses from nerve to nerve or nerve to muscle). What is the action of drugs such as tricyclic antidepressants (e.g. Imipramine) or selective serotonin reuptake inhibitors (SSRIs) (e.g. Citlaoprm or Sertroline) to exert their effect?

a. tricyclics:

b. SSRIs:

Answers

1. e) part of the peripheral nervous system responsible for involuntary controls such as thermoregulation or vasoconstriction.

2. a) true: *efferent is away (EXIT)*

   b) true

   c) false: *the dura mater is the outermost layer of the meninges. The inner is pia mater.*

   d) true: *eighth cranial nerve.*

3. a) pain.

4. a) cerebral cortex: 2

   b) corpus callosum: 1

   c) dermatome: 5

   d) white matter: 3

   e) myelin: 4

5. a) the end of a synapse when the NT is released, it is taken back up by the nerve cell to be repackaged and reused. In this case TCAs block the reuptake of serotonin and norepinephrine so the neurotransmitter stays (temporarily) in the gap between the nerves, called the synapse, to continue activating the post-synaptic cell. Since this is a broad acting drug it causes side effects related to norepinephrine and acetylcholine imbalances: involuntary muscle movements, secretions and digestion. They also block the effects of histamine which can lead to effects such as drowsiness, blurred vision, dry mouth, constipation and glaucoma.

   b) SSRIs: at the end of a synapse when the NT is released, it is taken back up by the nerve cell to be repackaged and reused. SSRIs prevents the reuptake of serotonin selectively in this case reducing the risk of side effects from other neurotransmitter effects.

Reflection: ask yourself

1. What do I know now that I didn't know before?

2. What am I confused/unclear about?

3. What areas do I need to focus on?

4. My action plan for further learning (make objectives SMART – (Specific/Measureable/Achievable/Realistic/Time-bound):

CHAPTER 2

Causes of alterations to level of consciousness

Tina Moore

Overview

An intact and fully operational brain is a requirement for a fully conscious state. Changes to levels of consciousness signify a developing brain dysfunction. Alterations to the level of consciousness is one of the early warning signs of physiological deterioration. Changes may be slight at first and challenging to recognise. Between the polarities of consciousness and unconsciousness there is a continuum of differing states of impaired consciousness (Blume et al., 2015). Transitory levels include drowsiness, confusion and comatose. Diagnosis of these levels is subjective.

Link to *Future Nurse Proficiencies* (NMC 2018)

Platform 3 Assessing needs and planning care (Section 3.2).
Annexe B, Part 1: Procedures for assessing people's needs for person-centred care. Specifically, 2.5: manage and interpret cardiac monitors, infusion pumps, blood glucose monitors and other monitoring devices and 2.10: measure and interpret blood glucose levels.

Expected knowledge

- Anatomy and physiology of central nervous system
- Reticular Activating System (RAS).

Introduction

There are various causes of alterations to the level of consciousness. These mainly fall into two categories – acute and chronic. Acute states of impaired consciousness are potentially reversible. Acute states are commonly caused by metabolic upsets such as hypoglycaemia or drug intoxication altering brain function but are usually reversible. Chronic states can frequently signal underlying brain damage and therefore are irreversible.

Content

Consciousness	Causes of alteration to level of consciousness	Blood glucose regulation
Hypoglycaemia	Hyperglycaemia	Blood Glucose Monitoring
Levels of impaired consciousness		

Learning outcomes

- Define consciousness
- Demonstrate knowledge and understanding of the different levels of impaired consciousness
- Show an understanding and list the causes of unconsciousness
- Correctly use equipment to monitor blood glucose.

Key background

A good marker for neurological changes and clinical deterioration is an alteration to the level of consciousness. Consciousness relates to a situation where the person is awake and has an awareness of their surroundings (the ability of the cerebral cortex to filter the sensory information received and then responding accordingly). Therefore a state of consciousness is not just being awake; the person is also responsive to stimuli such as sight and audio.

A fully conscious disposition requires an intact and totally functioning brain. Alterations to one's level of consciousness denote a progressing brain dysfunction. The term 'unconsciousness' has no one particular clinical definition. However, most recognised descriptions within clinical practice imply that the individual is oblivious of their environment and is unable to respond appropriately to verbal or painful stimuli.

The reticular formation, particularly the reticular activating system (RAS), is located in the brainstem. All sensory pathways link to the reticular formation. The RAS is a primitive network of interconnecting nerve cells and fibres that receives input from multiple sensory pathways. It controls the ability to be awake and sleep and receives input signals from the five senses (visual, auditory, touch, smell, taste).

The brain also auto-regulates its own blood flows which means that there is a constant flow between a mean arterial pressure of 60 mmHg and 150 mmHg (mean arterial pressure, or MAP, is the average blood pressure throughout the cardiac cycle). With a higher MAP, there is an increased blood flow and with a lower MAP there is a reduced blood flow. Alterations to the auto-regulation would indicate traumatic brain injury. In order to minimise problems with ischaemia, the patient's blood pressure should be maintained within normal parameters.

CONSCIOUSNESS/UNCONSCIOUSNESS

Consciousness is a function of the reticular formation (RF) which is located in the brainstem. All sensory pathways link into the RF. The Reticular Activating System (RAS) is a feature of the RF and is responsible for **arousal** from sleep (wakefulness) and maintaining consciousness and **awareness**. The arousal reaction is dependent on the stimulation of the RAS. The RAS receives input signals from a wide range of sources, including the senses (visual, auditory, touch, smell and taste).
Consciousness is a state of awareness of both their own self and their surroundings.

Unconsciousness is the physiological state where the patient is unaware for their surroundings and of themselves. Sudden loss of consciousness is an emergency situation and potentially life threatening due to the reduced airway reflexes that could lead to airway obstruction but as this is acute, can be reversible.

Conscious —— Unconscious

➢ Conscious: Alert and oriented
➢ Confused: Disoriented to time and place
➢ Somnolent: Drowsy, lethargic, sleepy
➢ Stuporous: Arousable with stimuli
➢ Obtunded: Cannot maintain arousal without repeated stimuli
➢ Comatose: Cannot be aroused and unresponsive with surroundings

Causes of alterations in level of consciousness

➢ **Metabolic** – Hepatic/ureaemic/hyperglycaemia/hypoglycaemia
➢ **Poisons/drugs** – sedatives, alcohol intoxication, cocaine
➢ **Increased brain volume** – tumours, cerebral oedema
➢ **Increased cerebral blood volume** – Haematoma caused by head trauma
➢ **Decreased cerebral metabolism** – hypoxaemia, hypercapnia, acidosis, alkalosis
➢ **Circulatory** – brain injury caused by hypoxaemia, ischaemia, shock, stroke
➢ **Infection** – systemic (sepsis) or cerebral (encephalitis, meningitis)
➢ **Haemorrhage** – cerebral, subarachnoid

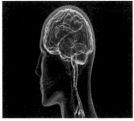

FIGURE 2.1 Consciousness/unconsciousness

BLOOD GLUCOSE REGULATION

Control of blood glucose is dependent upon effective metabolic processes. Glucose is essential to maintain brain, renal and erythrocyte energy sources. Insulin and glucagon are hormones responsible for carbohydrate metabolism and glucose control. Interference will upset homeostasis. Normal blood glucose level for someone without diabetes or ill health is 4.0–5.9 mmol/l (NICE 2020).

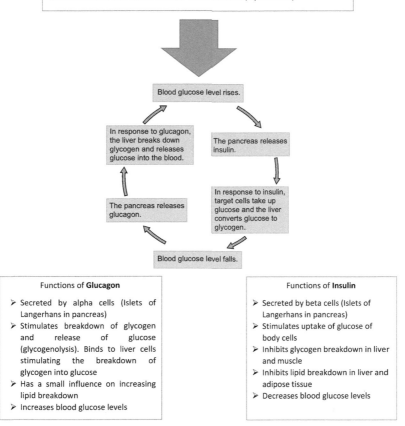

FIGURE 2.2 Blood glucose regulation

HYPOGLYCAEMIA

Hypoglycaemia is a situation when the blood glucose level is unable to meet the metabolic demands of the body. It results from an imbalance between glucose supply, glucose utilisation, and existing insulin concentration. It can result from aggressive insulin therapy used to treat hyperglycaemia. If conscious and able to swallow – fast acting carbohydrates. If unconscious – glucagon (if unsuitable or no response the glucose).

Hypoglycaemia can be defined as 'mild' (self-treatable) and 'severe'. Generally, inpatients with a blood-glucose concentration less than 4 mmol/litre should be treated (NICE 2020).

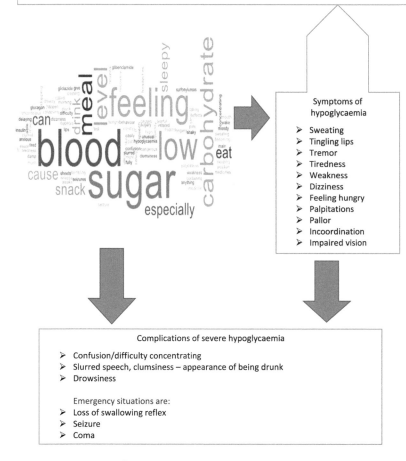

Symptoms of hypoglycaemia

➢ Sweating
➢ Tingling lips
➢ Tremor
➢ Tiredness
➢ Weakness
➢ Dizziness
➢ Feeling hungry
➢ Palpitations
➢ Pallor
➢ Incoordination
➢ Impaired vision

Complications of severe hypoglycaemia

➢ Confusion/difficulty concentrating
➢ Slurred speech, clumsiness – appearance of being drunk
➢ Drowsiness

Emergency situations are:
➢ Loss of swallowing reflex
➢ Seizure
➢ Coma

FIGURE 2.3 Hypoglycaemia

HYPERGLYCAEMIA

When insulin is deficient (type 2 diabetes) or absent (type 1 diabetes) blood glucose levels will remain high after a meal, during illness (including infection or acute illness) or stressful events or certain medication such as steroid therapy.

Hyperglycaemia = blood glucose is more than 7.0 mmol/l before a meal and 8.5 mmol/l after a meal (Diabetes UK 2020).

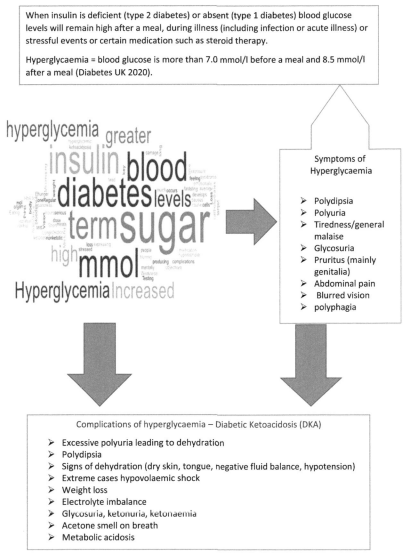

Symptoms of Hyperglycaemia

➢ Polydipsia
➢ Polyuria
➢ Tiredness/general malaise
➢ Glycosuria
➢ Pruritus (mainly genitalia)
➢ Abdominal pain
➢ Blurred vision
➢ polyphagia

Complications of hyperglycaemia – Diabetic Ketoacidosis (DKA)

➢ Excessive polyuria leading to dehydration
➢ Polydipsia
➢ Signs of dehydration (dry skin, tongue, negative fluid balance, hypotension)
➢ Extreme cases hypovolaemic shock
➢ Weight loss
➢ Electrolyte imbalance
➢ Glycosuria, ketonuria, ketonaemia
➢ Acetone smell on breath
➢ Metabolic acidosis

FIGURE 2.4 Hyperglycaemia

CAPILLARY BLOOD GLUCOSE (CBG) MONITORING

Capillary blood glucose monitoring provides an immediate and accurate indication of how the body is controlling glucose metabolism and provides feedback to guide the treatment adjustments in order to achieve optimum blood glucose levels.

Equipment
Blood glucose (BG) meter/test strips (in date)/control solution/single use safety lancets/disposable gloves /cotton wool or gauze/sharps box/tray for equipment

Follow manufacturer's instructions
Procedure

- Correct patient, explain procedure and gain consent. Place in comfortable position.
- Wash and dry hands before and after procedure.
- Check status of peripheries (numbness, pins and needles, circulation).
- Patient's skin should be clean and dry (wash hands with soap and warm water); do not use alcohol wipes.
- Discard any contaminated strips.
- Turn on BG meter and ensure it is collaborated.
- Put on gloves.
- Ensure correct depth setting of lancet is used for patient. Ensure site of piercing is rotated.
- Pierce the side or top if finger to obtain blood sample. Place drop of blood on strip.
- Insert testing strip into BG meter and read results.
- Dispose of lancet in sharps container.
- Place gauze over puncture site. Monitor for excessive bleeding.
- Document results and escalate where necessary.

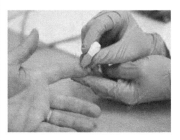

Finger piercing using a lancet

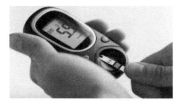

Blood glucose meter

Indications:	Contraindications (affecting the accuracy of results)	Principles of CBG monitoring
• Diabetes diagnosis • Monitor and manage diabetes • Acute management of hyper/hypoglycaemia from diabetes or primary illness • Monitor side effects of steroid therapy and total parenteral nutrition	• Peripheral vascular failure – dehydration/poor peripheral circulation • Pre-eclampsia • Some renal dialysis treatments • Hyperlipidaemia	• Severe consequences if not preformed accurately • Frequency of monitoring will be dependent upon patient needs

FIGURE 2.5 Capillary blood glucose monitoring

Activity: now test yourself

1. Which of the following is **not** an altered level of consciousness?

   a) confusion

   b) somnolence

   c) stuporous

   d) obtunded

   e) coma.

2. Name five pathophysiological causes of alteration to level of consciousness.

3. **True** or **false**? Sweating tiredness, dizziness, incoordination are all signs of hyperglycaemia.

4. **True** or **false**? Dehydration and hypovolaemic shock are key complications of hyperglycaemia.

5. Capillary blood glucose monitoring – what assessment of the peripheries should be undertaken before the procedure?

   a) numbness, pins and needles, nail varnish

   b) numbness, pins and needles, dullness

   c) numbness, pins and needles, circulation

   d) numbness, pins and needles, paraesthesia.

Answers

1. None – they are all examples of altered level of consciousness.

2. Any of the following:

   metabolic

   poisons/drugs

   increased brain volume

   increased cerebral blood volume

   decreased cerebral metabolism

   circulatory

   infection

   haemorrhage.

3. False. *They are all signs of hypoglycaemia.*

4. True, due to osmotic diuresis caused by considerably high blood glucose levels.

5. c) numbness, pins and needles, circulation. *'Paraesthesia' is another term for pins and needles; 'dullness' is another term for numbness.*

Reflection: ask yourself

1 What do I know now that I didn't know before?

2. What am I confused/unclear about?

3. What areas do I need to focus on?

4. My action plan for further learning (make objectives SMART – Specific/Measurable/Achievable/Realistic/Time-bound):

CHAPTER 3

Neurological assessment

Tina Moore

Overview

Neurological assessment is a good indicator of associated neurological changes with clinical deterioration. Not only can the neurological assessment determine subtle and rapid change in the patient's condition, it can also help to detect life-threatening situations and deterioration and establish the extent of injury for those with head trauma.

It is an aid in the diagnosis of neurological deficit and the measurement of progress. Assessing level of consciousness is a key area in the NEWS2 scoring system for recognising acute illness and physiological deterioration.

Link to *Future Nurse Proficiencies* (NMC 2018)

Platform 3 Assessing needs and planning care (Section 3.5).

Annexe B, Part 1: Procedures for assessing people's needs for person-centred care. Specifically, 2.1: take, record and interpret vital signs manually and via technological devices; 2.12 undertake, respond to and interpret neurological observations and assessments; and 2.13 identify and respond to signs of deterioration and sepsis.

Expected knowledge

- Cranial nerves
- Taking and recording vital signs
- The requirements of consciousness
- Different levels of consciousness/unconsciousness
- Reasons for altered level of consciousness.

Introduction

Level of consciousness is a good indicator of neurological changes and clinical deterioration. A neurological assessment should provide the means for diagnosis of neurological deficit and the measurement of progress as it is considered essential in the assessment of acutely ill patients (NICE, 2007, Resuscitation Council UK, 2015). Though 'simple' to use, the GCS is a complex tool and should be used by experienced practitioners (although this assessment is often delegated to student nurses who are junior and inexperienced in using the tool, increasing the risk of misinterpretation). The GCS should be used with patients who are not alert or have head trauma.

Accuracy of assessment is crucial. To identify discrepancies with assessment it is suggested that at shift handover assessment of the patient's GCS is conducted together by nurses on both shifts.

Content

Cranial Nerves	Assessment of level of consciousness	Assessment of mental status
Limb movements	Cushing's response	Pupil reaction
Lumbar puncture		

Learning outcomes

- Demonstrate knowledge and understanding of the 12 cranial nerves and how to assess them
- Describe the rationale for undertaking an assessment of level of consciousness
- Correctly assess level of consciousness
- Correctly perform the skill of assessing pupil reaction
- Recognise signs and symptoms of Cushing's response.

Key background

The Glasgow Coma Scale (GCS) offers a standardised, consistent approach to assessing the level of consciousness. The GCS directly assesses the functioning of the brainstem and demonstrates to the assessor that the reticular activating system has been stimulated and the patient is aware of their environment. As a neurological assessment tool, it can provide a basic mechanism for the diagnosis of neurological deficit and the means for measuring progress. It can also provide and essential base line for comparison. The GCS has also been used as a prognostic device during immediate assessment following a head injury. The lower the score, the poorer the prognosis.

This is achieved by appraising three behavioural responses: **eye opening (E)**; **verbal response (V)**; **motor response (M)**. The lowest score achievable is 3 (total unresponsiveness), while the maximum is 15 (awake, alert and fully responsive). A score of less than 8 is acknowledged to be meaningful as it is associated with the patient's airway potentially becoming compromised due to unconsciousness, and thus requires instant and appropriate airway management (in some instances this may mean electively ventilating the patient). Similarly, a decrease in the motor score by one or an overall deterioration of two is also meaningful and must be reported (NICE, 2007). It is worthy to note that the GCS should not be used in isolation of a complete assessment of the patient.

It is important to take note that the GCS scoring may indeed be misleading in those patients who are hypoxaemic, haemodynamically unstable, having seizures (or post-ictal, i.e. post-seizure), showing little response or under the influence of sedation, alcohol or drug intoxication. In addition, eye opening is not always an indication of intact neurological functioning. Patients in a persistent vegetative state (PVS) will open their eyes (they can also track movement) as a direct reflect action generated by the RAS. This should be analysed within the context of their condition. It is also important to re-evaluate once any underlying acute condition has been corrected.

It is extremely difficult to accurately assess infants and children under the age of five using the GCS, and particularly those following head trauma. Therefore the recommendation from NICE (2020) is that such observations should be performed by experienced staff.

A quick judgement of the severity of dysfunction for the individual patient can be gained through the use of the total GCS score, which describes their level of consciousness. The disadvantage is that it provides less information than is presented by the three responses individually and is likely to be worthless if one component of the scale is not able to be tested. This tool should not be used in isolation. It is good practice to accompany the scores with written commentary (described in simple, objective terms to convey a clear, unambiguous picture of their responsiveness) of the assessment. Reasons for this are discussed later in the chapter. Despite this, it is important NOT to adapt the assessment findings to fit the patients – nurses must record what is seen/heard (without interpretation) but should accompany the score with descriptive assessment information.

Motor dysphasia causes the patient to be unable to say the words they wish to say. Expressive dysphasia may occur with a stroke. This is where the patient has difficulty putting words together to make meaning but may have comprehension.

It is critical that the assessment of level of consciousness using the GCS is performed accurately. To identify discrepancies with assessment, it is suggested that at shift handover assessment of the patient's GCS is conducted together by nurses on both shifts.

Any changes in pupil reaction, shape or size are usually a late sign of raised intracranial pressure (ICP) especially succeeding head trauma. Sluggish or suddenly dilated unequal pupils are a sign that oedema or haematoma is worsening and the oculomotor cranial nerve is being compressed (herniated) through the foramen magnum. 'Blown pupils' (large and unreactive to light) follow herniation of part of the temporal lobe through the foramen magnum. The use of eye drops such as atropine can dilate pupils.

In relation to the regularity of monitoring observations, NICE (2020) suggests that these should be taken and recorded on a half-hourly basis until a GCS equal to 15 has been achieved. The minimum frequency of observations for patients with a GCS equal to 15 should be, starting after the initial assessment in the emergency department, as follows:

Half-hourly for two hours. Then once hourly for four hours. Then two hourly thereafter. Should the patient with a GCS equal to 15 deteriorate at any time after the initial two-hour period, observations should revert to half-hourly and follow the original frequency schedule. Needless to say, each patient should be individually assessed for the need to deviate from this guidance.

CRANIAL NERVES

I **Olfactory** – sensory function – smell (to test – block one nostril and get patient to smell something non-toxic and distinctive e.g. lemon, coffee.

II **Optic** – sensory function – visual (to test – use pen torch, note pupil size, shape and symmetry). Information to the brain (test visual acuity via the Smellen chart (like the one in an optician), using an ophthalmoscope to assess the optic disc (training required)). Pupillary reflexes (discussed in Figure 3.4)

III **Oculomotor** – motor function controlling eye movement and eyelid function. Observe for ptosis and strabismus. Hold your finger or pen upwards, ask patient to follow your finger with their eyes, keeping their head still.

IV **Trochlear** – motor function for eye movement downward/inward (same test as Oculomotor). Observe for double vision.

V **Trigeminal** – sensory and motor function. Facial sensation and mastication (to test – light touch to patient's sternum first (benchmark) then they should close their eyes and say each time you touch their face with the same pressure). Corneal reflex is also a test associated with this nerve.

VI **Abducens** – motor function eye movement (muscle) problems can cause a squint.

VII **Facial** – motor and sensory functions. Facial expressions and taste. Facial expressions and movement should be symmetrical. Monitor for unilateral weakness (facial drooping).

VIII **Vestibulocochlear** (auditory) – sensory sound and balance from inner ear to brain. Assess hearing, balance.

IX **Glossopharyngeal** – motor and sensory functions. Involved in swallowing, taste and phonation.

X **Vagus** – motor and sensory functions. Senses aortic blood pressure, slows heart rate, stimulates digestive organs (test gag reflex, swallowing).

XI **Accessory** – motor function – sternocleidomastoid and trapezius muscles (test – shoulder movement/shrug, head rotation).

XII **Hypoglossal** motor function. Tongue movement (test – protrude tongue, push tongue in cheek).

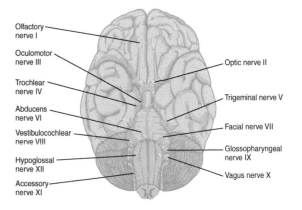

FIGURE 3.1 Cranial nerves

ASSESSMENT OF LEVEL OF CONSCIOUSNESS

The Glasgow Coma Scale (GCS) assesses the level of consciousness. It is 'simple' to use, but is a complex tool and should be used by experienced practitioners or at the very least under their supervision. The GCS should be used with all patients who are not alert or have head trauma.

ACVPU
A – Alert and oriented. Do not ask questions that provide a 'yes/no' answer. Ask the patient simple open ended questions in relation to time, place and person.
C – Confusion
V – Responds to verbal stimulus.
P – Responds to pain – note if patient moans or withdraws from the stimulus.
U – Unresponsive.

Best motor response – the most reliable predictor of prognosis.
Obeys commands (6M) obeys simple commands. *Localises to central pain* (5M) Patient tries to remove source of pain e.g. pressure source or pulling of the oxygen mask/nasogastric tube. *Withdrawal from pain* (4M) Bends arm at the elbow towards source of pain but fails to locate source. Assess both arms independently. *Abnormal flexion to pain* (3M) Flexes/bends the arms towards trunk. There is also internal rotation and adduction of the shoulder and flexion of the elbow. Reaction is slower.
Extension to pain (2M) Elbow and internal shoulder is straight and wrist internal rotation occur. Poorer prognosis.
No response (1M) to painful stimuli.

Best eye response – assesses brainstem and reticular activating system function (inform the patient what is to be done, apologise for the need to hurt them).
• *Eyes open spontaneously* (E4). Do NOT talk (automatically reduces score to E3).
• *Eyes open to speech* (E3)
• *Eyes open in response to pain only* (E2) – gently shake or touch the shoulder first. Then gradually increase the nature of the pressure.
Peripheral pressure – Pen pressed to the lateral outer aspect of the second or third finger, NOT on actual nail bed (damage to nailbed). Rotate the point of pressure on each assessment.
Central stimuli – Trapezius squeeze (preferred approach). Hold trapezius muscle between thumb and forefingers for a maximum of 10 seconds. Note verbal or non-verbal responses. Gradually increase pressure if indicated.
Supra-orbital pressure – only use when trained to do this correctly. Pressure is applied through the flat of the thumb on the supra-orbital ridge under the eyebrow pressing on the facial nerve, graduating pressure for approximately thirty seconds. Omit if there is any orbital damage or skull fracture.
Sternal rub and mandibular pressure are inappropriate for repeated assessments.
No response (E1) before scoring, ensure adequacy of painful stimuli. If eyes are closed, swollen, facial fractures or dressings – this is recorded as 'C' (closed) on the chart, scoring E1.

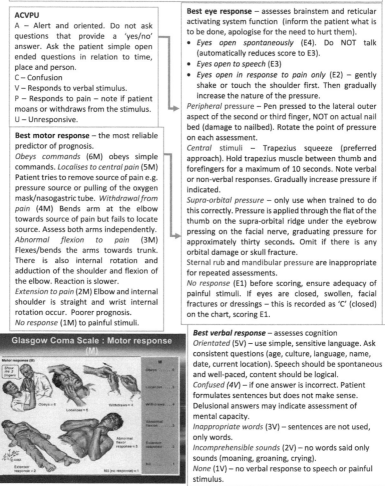

Glasgow Coma Scale : Motor response (M)

Best verbal response – assesses cognition
Orientated (5V) – use simple, sensitive language. Ask consistent questions (age, culture, language, name, date, current location). Speech should be spontaneous and well-paced, content should be logical.
Confused (4V) – if one answer is incorrect. Patient formulates sentences but does not make sense. Delusional answers may indicate assessment of mental capacity.
Inappropriate words (3V) – sentences are not used, only words.
Incomprehensible sounds (2V) – no words said only sounds (moaning, groaning, crying).
None (1V) – no verbal response to speech or painful stimulus.

FIGURE 3.2 Assessment of level of consciousness

ASSESSING MENTAL STATUS

Mini-Mental State Examination (MMSE)

Patient's Name: _____   Date: _____

Instructions: Score one point for each correct response within each question or activity.

Maximum Score	Patient's Score	Questions
5		"What is the year? Season? Date? Day? Month?"
5		"Where are we now? State? County? Town/city? Hospital? Floor?"
3		The examiner names three unrelated objects clearly and slowly, then the instructor asks the patient to name all three of them. The patient's response is used for scoring. The examiner repeats them until patient learns all of them, if possible.
5		"I would like you to count backward from 100 by sevens." (93, 86, 79, 72, 65, ...) Alternative: "Spell WORLD backwards." (D-L-R-O-W)
3		"Earlier I told you the names of three things. Can you tell me what those were?"
2		Show the patient two simple objects, such as a wristwatch and a pencil, and ask the patient to name them.
1		"Repeat the phrase: 'No ifs, ands, or buts.'"
3		"Take the paper in your right hand, fold it in half, and put it on the floor." (The examiner gives the patient a piece of blank paper.)
1		"Please read this and do what it says." (Written instruction is "Close your eyes.")
1		"Make up and write a sentence about anything." (This sentence must contain a noun and a verb.)
1		"Please copy this picture." (The examiner gives the patient a blank piece of paper and asks him/her to draw the symbol below. All 10 angles must be present and two must intersect.)
30		TOTAL

General appearance – is the patient able to look after themselves (personal hygiene, clothing)?
Behaviour – ability to build a rapport, use of eye contact, facial expression (e.g. sad, angry), over exaggeration, restless, abnormal movements (e.g. rocking, lip smacking, tremors, involuntary movements)
Speech – rapid, slow, incoherent, slurred, minimal speaking, rambling, stammer, stutter, volume (very loud or very quiet)
Mood – subject assessment – low mood, anxiety, angry, enraged, sadness, hostility, euphoric, guilty, apathetic
Range and mobility of emotional expression:
Fixed – no change of emotion
Restricted – slight change of emotion
Labile – exaggerated changes – no control over emotions
Heightened/tense emotions (mania disorders)
Blunted/flat emotions (depression)
Congruence – emotions correspondence with thoughts
Incongruence – emotions not corresponding with thoughts
Thoughts – speed of thoughts, congruency of thoughts
Delusions – abnormal fixation
Obsession – irrational
Compulsion – repetitive compelled thoughts
Overvalued ideas – dominating thoughts
Suicidal thoughts
Homicidal/violent thoughts
Perception – hallucinations
Cognition – mental action or process of acquiring knowledge and understanding
Insight – ability to understand there is an issue
Judgement – ability to make considered decisions

FIGURE 3.3 Assessing mental status

CUSHING'S RESPONSE & PUPIL REACTION

Cushing's response

Vital Signs
Blood pressure – hypertension is part of the Cushing's response (the physiological response of brain swelling and raised intracranial pressure. Monitor very closely the trend of observations.
Heart rate – bradycardia demonstrates signs of raised intracranial pressure (Cushing's response).
Respiration – with raised intracranial pressure, a reduced respiratory rate will occur which is also irregular (loss of brainstem functioning). This is the third part of the Cushing's response.
Temperature – control centre in the hypothalamus (brainstem). Pyrexia occurs when thermoregulation fails.

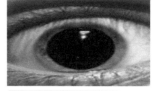

Dilated pupil

Pen torch with pupil sizes

Pupil reaction – assesses the 2nd (optic) and 3rd (oculomotor) cranial nerves.
Procedure for pupil reaction

1. Best conducted in a darkened area (where possible) with a bright shining pen torch.
2. Instruct patient not to look directly at light (artificial or direct). You may need to darken the room.
3. Patient's eyes should be open/eyelids held open.
4. With bright shining torch light on, gradually move it from the outside (head) towards the pupil.
5. Note pupil final size, shape and reaction to light in both eyes (brisk, sluggish, no reaction).
6. Normal pupil size is considered to be approximately 2–5mm. Normal shape is spherical and mid position.
7. Cataract, eye injuries, false eye, medication (opiates, barbiturates) can influence results.

'C' = closed eye (swelling or dressings). Record brisk pupils as '+' and unreactive pupils as '.' 'S' = sluggish.

Limb movements

➤ Ask patient to hold arms out in front of them for 20–30 seconds. Observe for signs of weakness or 'drifting' downwards.
➤ Put your hands palm to palm with patient–instruct patient to push and pull against your hands.
➤ Ask patient to lay on their bed. Instruct them to flex their knee and rest their foot on the bed. They should keep their foot on the bed whilst you try to straighten the leg. Then ask patient to straighten their leg and you provide resistance.

FIGURE 3.4 Cushing's response and pupil reaction

LUMBAR PUNCTURE

Lumbar puncture is the procedure to obtain cerebrospinal fluid (CSF) from the subarachnoid space in the lumbar region. It involves local anaesthesia. This procedure should NOT be performed on patients with raised intracranial pressure due to the high risk of coning (herniation of brainstem tissue through the foramen magnum). Any signs of infection around the proposed puncture site should also be a reason not to perform this procedure.

It is a specialist skill that requires specialist training. Your role as a student nurse is to assist in the procedure and to support and monitor the patient.

Reasons for a lumbar puncture:

➤ Obtain a sample of CSF for diagnosis – e.g. meningitis, Guillain Barrié syndrome.
➤ Introduce radio-opaque fluid into the subarachnoid space.
➤ Identify presence of blood in CSF (trauma or suspected subarachnoid haemorrhage).
➤ Identify raised ICP.
➤ Introduce intrathecal medication e.g. chemotherapy, antibiotics, anaesthesia.
➤ Insert Xray medium for myelogram.

Contraindications (NICE 2012)

➤ Signs of raised intracranial pressure
➤ Shock
➤ Extensive spreading purpura
➤ Unstable seizures
➤ Coagulation abnormalities
➤ Superficial infection at lumbar puncture site
➤ Respiratory insufficiency
➤ Significant degeneration joint disease
➤ Previous back surgery (hardware in place)

Procedure – this is performed by a doctor.

Equipment
PPE/trolley/sterile dressing pack with drapes/lumbar puncture pack /spinal manometer/two-way tap/antiseptic cleaning solution/local anaesthetic/sterile dressing/3 sterile specimen containers

1. Help to explain procedure to patient. Check consent has been signed.
2. Maintain privacy and dignity.
3. Help patient to get into and maintain appropriate position (normally laying on side, head neck flexed and knees drawn up to abdomen). Maximise safety.
4. Help prepare sterile field, maintaining asepsis.
5. Continually monitor patient throughout the procedure for adverse reactions.
6. Help patient to maintain a still position.
7. Help expose lumber region.
8. Hold sterile containers to receive the flow of CSF as instructed buy the doctor.
9. Apply pressure to site when needle has been removed. Cover with sterile dressing.
10. Patient to be placed in a comfortable position once completed.
11. Monitor patient's level of consciousness and vital signs.
12. Document procedure and patient's observations.
13. Arrange for specimens to be sent to the laboratory.

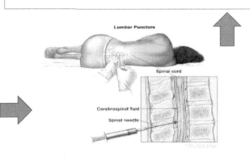

FIGURE 3.5 Lumbar puncture

Activity: now test yourself

1. Name eight of the 12 cranial nerves and their function.

2. What are the three components of the Glasgow Coma Scale that assesses level of consciousness?

3. **True** or **false**? Assessment of consciousness is a vital sign and is an early warning sign of a patient's clinical deterioration.

4. Cushing's response is:

   a) decreased blood pressure/increased heart rate/ decreased respiratory rate

   b) increased blood pressure/increased heart rate/ increased respiratory rate

   c) increased blood pressure/decreased heart rate/ increased respiratory rate

   d) increased blood pressure/decreased heart rate/ decreased respiratory rate.

Answers

1. Any of the following:

    I   Olfactory (smell)

    II   Optic (pupillary reflexes)

    III   Oculomotor (eye movement and eyelid function)

    IV   Trochlear (eye movement, downward/inward)

    V   Trigeminal (facial sensation and mastication)

    VI   Abducens (eye movement)

    VII   Facial (facial expressions and taste)

    VIII Vestibulocochlear (auditory)

    IX   Glossopharyngeal (swallowing, taste and phonation)

    X   Vagus (senses aortic blood pressure, slows heart rate, stimulates digestive organs)

    XI   Accessory (sternocleidomastoid and trapezius muscles)

    XII   Hypoglossalt (tongue movement).

2. Best eye response/best verbal response/best motor response.

3. True.

4. d) increased blood pressure/decreased heart rate/decreased respiratory rate.

Reflection: ask yourself

1. What do I know now that I didn't know before?

2. What am I confused/unclear about?

3. What areas do I need to focus on?

4. My action plan for further learning (make objectives SMART – Specific/Measurable/Achievable/Realistic/Time-bound):

CHAPTER 4

Caring for the unconscious patient

Tina Moore

Overview

Caring for the unconscious patient is not only confined to the practices of critical care and theatre nurses; unconsciousness can occur in any area of nursing. Causes of unconsciousness (acute and chronic) have been discussed in earlier chapters but the fundamental needs and care for someone who is unconscious is the same irrespective of the underlying cause.

Link to *Future Nurse Proficiencies* (NMC 2018)

Platform 3 Assessing needs and planning care (Section 3.5).

Annexe B, Part 1: Procedures for assessing people's needs for person-centred care. Specifically, 2.7: undertake a whole body systems assessment including respiratory, circulatory, neurological, musculoskeletal, cardiovascular and skin status; 2.8: undertake chest auscultation and interpret findings; 2.10: measure and interpret blood glucose levels; 2.12: undertake, respond to and interpret neurological observations and assessment; and 2.13: identify and respond to signs of deterioration and sepsis.

Annexe B, Part 2: Procedures for the planning, provision and management of person-centred nursing care. Specifically, 4: Use evidence-based, best practice approaches for meeting the needs for care and support with hygiene and the maintenance of skin integrity, accurately assessing the person's capacity for independence and self-care and initiating appropriate interventions; 5: Use evidence-based, best practice approaches for meeting needs for care and support with nutrition and hydration, accurately assessing the person's capacity for independence and self-care and initiating appropriate interventions; 6: Use evidence-based, best practice approaches for meeting needs for care and support with bladder and bowel health, accurately assessing the person's capacity for independence and self-care and initiating appropriate interventions; 7: Use evidence-based, best practice approaches for meeting needs for care and support with mobility and safety, accurately assessing the person's capacity for independence and self-care and initiating appropriate interventions; and 9: Use evidence-based, best practice approaches for meeting needs for care and support with the prevention and management of infection, accurately assessing the person's capacity for independence and self-care and initiating appropriate interventions.

Expected knowledge

- Your own beliefs and attitudes towards caring for a patient who is unconscious
- Fundamentals of airway management, fluid and hydration, elimination, skin care, hygiene care, communication and psychosocial care.

Introduction

Complete care of an unconscious patient presents a special challenge to nurses because the patient is totally dependent on the nurse's knowledge, skill and caring attitude for their safety and comfort needs. It is a legal and professional duty of the nurse to meeting these demands (NMC 2018).

Priorities include:

- Establishing and managing a clear airway
- Assessing level of consciousness
- Recording and evaluating vital signs
- Maintaining fluid and electrolyte balance
- Performing nursing care as appropriate to the patient's condition.

If appropriate, involve relatives and/or significant others in the care of the patient. When caring for the unconscious patient, even basic nursing care becomes a complex task. Much of the care required correlates with essential nursing procedures;

therefore only special considerations in relation to the unconscious patient will be discussed in this chapter.

Content

Airway management	Nutrition and hydration	Immobility – position/skin
Elimination – catheter	Hygiene	Psychosocial needs

Learning outcomes

- Identify the needs of the unconscious patient
- Demonstrate the ability to prioritise patient care, recognising the skills required for the assessment, planning and implementation of nursing care.

Key background

Unconsciousness is potentially life-threatening, since such patients have reduced airway reflexes and are considered unable to protect their own airway from aspiration or obstruction. When this occurs, it is an emergency situation and immediate intervention is required. If the patient is unconscious through alcohol intoxication there is a high risk of vomiting (potential to block the airway). With the patient vomiting or producing a lot of secretions from the mouth (e.g. fluid), there is always a risk of aspiration. If this occurs, patient management becomes more complex and risky. Noisy breathing (e.g. snoring) may indicate partial airway obstruction.

The medical management of the patient will be dependent upon the underlying cause of unconsciousness. For example, in the case of hypoxaemia, oxygen therapy; for diabetic ketoacidosis, aggressive fluid therapy; for seizures, medication such as phenytoin.

Oropharyngeal airway (do not use with mandibular or oral trauma) or nasopharyngeal (use with caution in patients with head trauma) airways may help prevent airway obstruction and can easily allow the removal of secretions via suctioning.

Once the airway remains clear, then promoting adequate ventilation is the next nursing priority. Any dentures should be removed and any loose teeth/crowns should be documented (these could be a source of airway obstruction if dislodged).

The supine position is not ideal as it generally causes a reduction in the residual volume and functional residual capacity of the lungs leading to possible atelectasis. Continuous oxygen saturation monitoring should be performed with frequent assessment of the patient's respiratory status.

Close monitoring of blood pressure and pulse is also required, not only to observe for signs of dehydration or for signs of increased intracranial pressure in a patient with head trauma but for increased cardiac workload and central fluid shifts from the legs to the thorax and head, which is a side effect of immobility.

As the patient will require supplementary nutrition and hydration, regular blood and urine tests should be performed in order to monitor electrolyte and metabolic changes. During a period of unconsciousness, nitrogen is lost from the body during the breakdown of protein, which can create a catabolic situation where nitrogen loss exceeds supply, meaning that muscle breakdown will occur. In severe cases, this includes the breakdown of intercostal muscles used for breathing. To assess the patient's protein needs, a 24-hour urine collection should also be undertaken.

It is extremely important that the patient is spoken to before being touched, just to reassure them that someone is there. Nurses should verbally reassure patients and talk them through procedures before starting them.

Therapeutic use of touch should be combined with kind and comforting words. However, this does need to be assessed individually as touch can also be perceived as invasive or at the very least threatening.

Complications can include:

- Airway obstruction
- Chest infection, atelectasis (partial collapse of the lung)
- Venous thromboembolism (deep vein thrombosis, pulmonary embolism)
- Muscle wasting
- Hyperglycaemia (caused by immobility)
- Irregular bowel activity (loose stool, constipation)
- Urinary incontinence/urinary infections
- Compromised skin integrity
- Poor hygiene (skin, feet, nails, teeth, ears, hair, eyes)
- Psychosocial needs going unmet.

AIRWAY MANAGEMENT

The unconscious patient lacks many vital and protective reflexes and depends on others for protection and maintenance of vital functions. It is a legal and professional duty of the nurse to ensure that the patient's safety is maintained during this critical period.

Causes of obstruction in the unconscious patient

➤ Tongue – poor positioning (most common cause)
➤ Foreign body (dislocated tooth)
➤ Fluid (vomit e.g. alcohol intoxication)
➤ Swelling/oedema of the face. throat, tongue (allergic reaction)
➤ Swelling/inflammatory processes (burns/smoke)
➤ Displacement of artificial airway adjuncts.

Maintaining a clear airway

➤ Remove dentures and note any loose teeth, caps (if possible these should be removed)
➤ Suctioning may be indicated for removal of fluid in the pharynx and mouth
➤ Use of airway adjunct
➤ Lateral position (see mobility mind map)

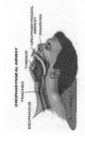

Oral pharyngeal airway (unconscious and no gag reflex). To measure – flange aligned to centre of lips, tip to angle of jaw. Insert 'upside down'.

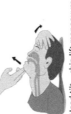

Head tilt – chin lift manoeuvre

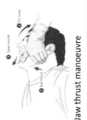

Jaw thrust manoeuvre

Signs of airway obstruction

Patency occurs when the patient is speaking clearly without distress.

Signs would include partial tracheal tug; irritability and agitation; reduced level of consciousness. DO NOT rely on cyanosis or reduced oxygen saturation levels as these are VERY late signs.

Partial obstruction (noises)

➤ Snoring (pharynx is partially obstructed by soft palate or tongue).
➤ Gurgling (fluid in the upper airway e.g. vomitus, sputum).
➤ Stridor (a harsh high pitch noise), commonly occurring on inspiration (caused by blockage above or at the level of the larynx) or expiratory (caused by bronchospasm).

Complete obstruction

➤ No breath sounds.
➤ Paradoxical chest and abdominal movements ('see-saw' respiration).

FIGURE 4.1 Airway management

NUTRITION AND HYDRATION

Enteral feeding via a nasogastric tube is normally the route to provide the nutrition required for the unconscious patient.

This can provide both short and long term solutions for nutritional problems. As the unconscious patient does not have 'cough or gag' reflexes, nurses should NOT be inserting the nasogastric tube. This will be the role of a doctor or anaesthetist. The nasogastric route is for short term solutions.

This is to prevent aspiration of stomach contents into the lungs – if this happens, there can be fatal consequences for the patient.

A rest period should be incorporated into the feeding regime to allow for gastric acidity to return to its normal level and in doing so reducing the risks of bacterial colonisation.

For longer term feeding a percutaneous endoscopic gastrostomy (PEG) tube is normally used.

➢ Monitor urea and electrolyte levels.
➢ 24-hour urine collection for assessing protein levels (muscle breakdown can occur when protein is broken down in body).
➢ Monitoring glucose levels (immobility can cause glucose intolerance). Insulin regime may be required to maintain adequate glucose levels.
➢ Monitor for signs of complications e.g. rhinitis, oesophageal irritation and gastritis.

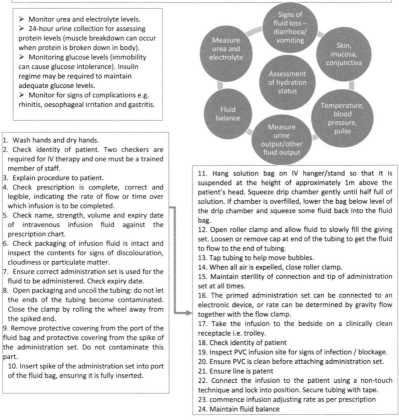

1. Wash hands and dry hands.
2. Check identity of patient. Two checkers are required for IV therapy and one must be a trained member of staff.
3. Explain procedure to patient.
4. Check prescription is complete, correct and legible, indicating the rate of flow or time over which infusion is to be completed.
5. Check name, strength, volume and expiry date of intravenous infusion fluid against the prescription chart.
6. Check packaging of infusion fluid is intact and inspect the contents for signs of discolouration, cloudiness or particulate matter.
7. Ensure correct administration set is used for the fluid to be administered. Check expiry date.
8. Open packaging and uncoil the tubing: do not let the ends of the tubing become contaminated. Close the clamp by rolling the wheel away from the spiked end.
9. Remove protective covering from the port of the fluid bag and protective covering from the spike of the administration set. Do not contaminate this part.
10. Insert spike of the administration set into port of the fluid bag, ensuring it is fully inserted.

11. Hang solution bag on IV hanger/stand so that it is suspended at the height of approximately 1m above the patient's head. Squeeze drip chamber gently until half full of solution. If chamber is overfilled, lower the bag below level of the drip chamber and squeeze some fluid back into the fluid bag.
12. Open roller clamp and allow fluid to slowly fill the giving set. Loosen or remove cap at end of the tubing to get the fluid to flow to the end of tubing.
13. Tap tubing to help move bubbles.
14. When all air is expelled, close roller clamp.
15. Maintain sterility of connection and tip of administration set at all times.
16. The primed administration set can be connected to an electronic device, or rate can be determined by gravity flow together with the flow clamp.
17. Take the infusion to the bedside on a clinically clean receptacle i.e. trolley.
18. Check identity of patient
19. Inspect PVC infusion site for signs of infection / blockage.
20. Ensure PVC is clean before attaching administration set.
21. Ensure line is patent
22. Connect the infusion to the patient using a non-touch technique and lock into position. Secure tubing with tape.
23. commence infusion adjusting rate as per prescription
24. Maintain fluid balance

FIGURE 4.2 Nutrition and hydration

ELIMINATION

Equipment: a 'catheter pack' (sterile drape/cotton gauze balls/gallipot/gauze surgical swabs/collecting receiver), plus: 2 x 10ml ampoules of 0.9% saline/urine collection bag (or urometer)/catheter (start with 12cH (short term use an uncoated latex, PVC, polytetrafluoroethylene (PTFE) or silver alloy catheter, longer term, use an all silicone, silicone elastomer or hydrogel coated catheter))/check for allergies/lidocaine (6 ml, 2%) gel/10ml ampoule of sterile water/10ml syringe and green needle/2 pairs of sterile gloves.

A urinary sheath may be used for a male patient.
Female catheterisation – requires 2 nurses.

1. Ensure privacy and dignity. Explain procedure to patient.
2. Wash and dry hands. Put on an apron.
3. Check for any allergies e.g. latex or anaesthetic gels. If allergic to latex, use a silicone catheter.
4. Open catheter pack, using aseptic technique, place the sterile field onto the top shelf of the trolley.
5. Open other packs onto sterile field now stretched out on the trolley, pour 0.9% saline into gallipot.
6. Place patient in supine position, knees bent and hips flexed. Separate feet placed flat on bed (60cm apart). Second nurse holds legs in position. Put protective sheet under their buttocks, adjust lighting.
7. Wash and dry hands.
8. Put on a pair of sterile gloves without contaminating the sterile field.
9. Hold labia open (exposing the urethral meatus) with your dominant hand for the remainder of the procedure. With other hand cleanse the urethral meatus, using saline soaked gauze balls. Use each gauze for a single downward movement (towards anus).
10. Insert nozzle of anaesthetic gel into urethra and squeeze gel. Allow 5 minutes for the anaesthetic to work. Place the sterile drape.
11. Put a little lubricating gel on tip of catheter. Place the collecting bowl for urine between the patient's legs.
12. Using the blue sterile sheath to hold the catheter, tear a small hole in the perforations near the tip, gently pass it into the urinary meatus.
13. Introduce the catheter into the urethral opening in an upward and backward direction. Advance the catheter until 5 or 6cm has been inserted and urine begins to flow then advance the catheter a further 1–2 cm, thus 6 to 8 cm in total). Never force the catheter if resistance is felt.
14. If no urine present, withdraw catheter and start procedure again.
15. Attach appropriate urine collecting product.
16. When the catheter is successfully placed inflate catheter balloon with 10 ml of sterile water Withdraw catheter slightly to ensure balloon is inflated and secure.

> Constipation has been frequently defined as failure to pass stool for 72 hours. Constipation and faecal impaction are common with patients who are immobile, critically ill or unconscious.
> Diseases in which there is a physiological change to some tissue or organ of the body (e.g., radiation therapy, inflammatory bowel disease, diabetes, stroke).
> Functional disorders, such as irritable bowel syndrome, intestinal obstructions.

Constipation can cause abdominal distension, vomiting, restlessness, gut obstruction, and at its worst perforation.
Hard, dry stool.
Infrequent defaecation. Irregular bowel pattern.
Distension, discomfort, and restlessness from constipation could explain failure to wean.

> Monitoring of bowel function (bowel chart).
> Ensure patient is well hydrated (unless there are contraindications e.g. chronic renal failure).
> Monitoring of medication e.g. opiates, diuretics.
> Use of laxatives, e.g. Senna, lactulose (where there is no contraindication).
> Rectal suppositories or enemas as a last resort.
> Manual evacuation as a last resort (this procedure can cause cardiac arrhythmias).

Bristol Stool Chart

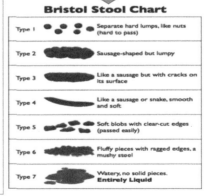

Type 1	Separate hard lumps, like nuts (hard to pass)
Type 2	Sausage-shaped but lumpy
Type 3	Like a sausage but with cracks on its surface
Type 4	Like a sausage or snake, smooth and soft
Type 5	Soft blobs with clear-cut edges (passed easily)
Type 6	Fluffy pieces with ragged edges, a mushy stool
Type 7	Watery, no solid pieces. Entirely Liquid

FIGURE 4.3 Elimination needs

IMMOBILITY

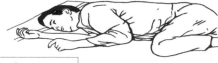

Risks factors for pressure injury/ulceration

- **Change in body weight distribution** – most of the body weight is distributed to the lateral aspect of the lower scapula, the lateral aspect of the ilium, and the greater trochanter of the femur, leading to:
- **Pressure to points on the dependent side of the body**, e.g. ears, shoulders, ribs, hips, knees and ankles, as well as brachial plexus injury, venous pooling, diminished lung capacity and DVT. A pressure-reducing or mattress or pillow / pressure relieving aids should be used as indicated.
- **Incontinence**
- **Perspiration**
- **Poor neutrino / dehydration**
- **Obesity**
- **Chronic illness (e.g. diabetes, respiratory, skin disorders, vascular disease)**
- **Extremes of age**
- **Medications (e.g. immunosuppressant)**

Interventions

- Use of an appropriate assessment and monitoring pressure injury risk tool.
- Avoid injuring the skin (moving and handling in accordance to approved techniques).
- Keep skin clean and dry.
- When drying skin use a patting technique (rubbing may damage the skin).
- Use of barrier creams.
- Use of pressure relieving mattress (NICE 2015).
- 2–4 hourly change of position (NICE 2015).
- Anti-embolism stockings/anticoagulants (subcutaneous).
- Passive limb movement (muscle atrophy).
- Body and neck in neutral alignment – preventing pressure ulcers, foot drop and contractures.

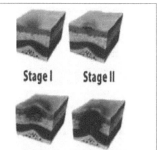

Stage 1 – **Intact skin.** Localised area of non-blanchable erythema (in dark skin the area will not look red but different to the rest of the skin). Purple / maroon changes may indicate deep tissue pressure injury. Avoid further skin damage.

Stage 2 – **Partial thickness loss.** May present as an abrasion or blister. Granulation tissue, slough or eschar are not present. Avoid further skin damage, protect the skin surrounding the wound. Apply dressings.

Stage 3 – **Full thickness loss.** Adipose tissue is visible in the ulcer, granulation (around edges), may be evidence of tunnelling of wound. Avoid further skin damage, regimented position changes, assessment of nutrition, pressure relieving aids. Absorbent dressings.

Stage 4. **Full thickness skin and tissue loss** – with exposed or directly palpable fascia, muscle, tendon, ligament, cartridge or bone. Treatment as per grade 3, infection treated with antibiotics, x-ray/scan to assess level of tissue/bone damage.

FIGURE 4.4 Immobility

PERSONAL HYGIENE – WASHING

Equipment needed at the bedside:
Two towels/own wash basin and hand
hot water/skin cleanser – soap or soap
substitute/shower gel/foam
wash/disposable wipes/wash cloth/non-
sterile gloves and apron/clean linen/slide
sheets/linen bag and rubbish bag/clean
clothing for the patient/moisturiser,
deodorant, make-up(if required).
Note religious and cultural practice of the
patient

Procedure – Preparation

1. Even though the patient is unconscious, explain the procedure to them.
2. Wash hands before and after procedure. Put on protective clothing as required (Standard Infection Control Procedures).
3. Remove top bedding covers, keeping the top sheet on the patient assist with removal of the patients clothing as necessary underneath the sheet.
4. For maintaining safety, patient should not be wearing any items of jewellery.
5. Once undressed keep the patient covered with the top sheet as this will ensure that the patient is kept warm and you continue to maintain privacy and dignity.

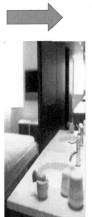

1. Remove any glasses or hearing aids.
2. Place a towel across patient's chest and wash face and neck area. using a disposable wipe and cleansing agent (if used), start with the eyelids first, then forehead, cheeks, nose, ears and jaw ending at the neck. Ensure that no soap/cleanser gets into the patient's eyes.
3. Rinse off any cleansing agent and gently pat face dry using the second towel.
4. Apply facial moisturiser (if used) then replace glasses/hearing aids.
5. Place a towel under the arm and using a new wipe and cleansing agent, wash arms one at a time and the chest.
6. Placing the towel under the arm and using a new wipe with preferred cleansing agent wash the whole of the arm from shoulder, armpit, fingertips.
7. Wash the arm furthest away first.
8. Rinse off the cleansing agent and pat dry using the second towel and repeat this for the next arm.
9. Once skin is dry apply deodorant if required.
10. Remove towel to expose the chest area to wash and rinse. Pay particular attention to underneath the female breasts, checking for any redness, ensuring the area is dried thoroughly. Cover patient to maintain dignity.
11. With assistance, roll patient onto side, place the towel along their back and buttocks. Wash and dry back area. Once completed replace top clothing.
12. Check skin on back for any redness especially the pressure points (e.g. shoulder blades, sacrum).
13. Patients with intravenous lines, put the bag and tubing in first through the sleeve, followed by the patient's arm. Hang the bag on the drip stand then put the other arm in the other sleeve and pull garment down covering the patient's torso.

1. Wash legs, one at a time (furthest away first).
2. Remove anti-embolic stockings if worn.
3. Place the towel under the leg, wash, rinse and dry the leg from the hip to the toes. Ensure that between the toes are washed and dried. Examine the condition of the skin. Check pressure points on heals.
4. Repeat the same for the other leg.
5. Take extra care and vigilance with patients who have diabetes, as they may develop the complication of peripheral neuropathy, where foot injuries do not heal very well.
6. Change water and disposable wipe and wash and dry the genital area.
7. For all female patients start from the pubic area working downwards to the labia and perineum also known as cleaning from front to back to minimise infection risk.
8. For male patients who are uncircumcised, clean the glans penis by gently pulling the foreskin back to clean the glans penis area. Dispose of wipes and water.
9. Change bottom sheet.
10. Place patient in lateral position.
11. Change the rest of the bedding.
12. Document any significant findings.

FIGURE 4.5 Hygiene needs

HAIR CARE AND EYE CARE

Hair Care

Equipment

2 x towels/jug/2 x large wash bowls (for water and a receptacle)/bedside table/shampoo and conditioner/comb/brush/optional hair dryer/incontinence pads/slide sheet/personal protective clothing

Procedure – 2 nurses or family member

1. Prepare all equipment and have within easy reach. Explain procedure. Maintain privacy and dignity.
2. Wash hands. Put on required protective clothing.
3. Water should be warm.
4. Pull bed away from the wall. Remove back rest to facilitate access to washing the patient's hair.
5. Adjust height of bed and position the bedside table behind the patient at the head of bed. Cover table with the incontinence pads; put the hair washing tray on the table and position receiving wash bowl beneath the drip outlet if required on the side.
6. Using the slide sheet, move patient up the bed (head is resting in the hair washing tray). MONITOR THE AIRWAY AT ALL TIMES.
7. Place one towel around the patient's chest and neck area. Ensure the patient's head is resting in the head washing tray to collect the water.
8. Assess condition of hair and scalp.
9. Using jug with water pour over patient's hair.
10. Apply shampoo and wash the hair and rinse thoroughly. If required, apply conditioner and rinse.
11. Wrap other towel around the patient's hair to dry. Move the patient back down the bed.
12. Continue to dry hair thoroughly, using the comb/brush and hair dryer (if available).
13. Tidy around the bed area; dispose of all equipment; decontaminate wash bowls, remove protective clothing and wash hands.
14. Ensure that the patient safe.

Eye Care

Equipment

Clean trolley/eye care pack or dressing pack which should have two gallipots (one for each eye) and lint free gauze/normal saline/apron and gloves/hand cleaning gel

Procedure

1. Explain procedure to the patient Maintain privacy and dignity.
2. Take a swab for any eye discharge.
3. Ensure easy access to eye.
4. Patient should not be wearing glasses/contact lenses.
5. Lay on back, ONLY if the patient can maintain their airway, otherwise leave patient in the lateral position.
6. Wash hands before and after. Have all equipment opened and prepared on the trolley.
7. Using the lint free gauze, moisten in normal saline and gently cleanse the upper eyelid of the first eye (from inner part of the closed eye (closest to the nose)) to the outer aspect in one movement and discard the gauze.
8. Repeat until eye is clean. Clean the upper eyelid first with eye closed from the inner aspect of the eye to the outer aspect.
9. Clean the lower eyelid (gently open eyelid), from the inner aspect outwards with one gentle movement and discard the gauze. Repeat until eye is clean.
10. Dry eye with a swabbing action from the inner to outer eye in one movement using dry lint free gauze.
11. Decontaminate hands. Change gloves.
12. Repeat procedure for the second eye.
13. Instil eye drops or artificial tears if prescribed.
14. Keep eyes shut to prevent drying (may be necessary to tape shut using hypo allergic tape).
15. Clear the trolley and dispose of all equipment, wash your hands.
16. Document care and findings.

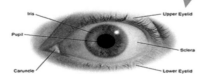

FIGURE 4.6 Hair care and eye care

ORAL CARE

Oral assessment

- Pain in the mouth?
- A sticky dry feeling in mouth and throat?
- Problems with taste?
- Breath that smells?
- Red, peeling, dry or cracked lips?
- Dry, inflamed, furry tongue. Any signs of ulceration or cracked tongue?
- Decay looking teeth, well-fitting dentures?
- Loose teeth (including children)?
- Inflamed mucous membranes of the gum. Sings of bleeding or blisters?
- Thick white patches on mucous membranes and tongue?
- Dentures – remove.
- Loose teeth/crowns – note or remove if possible.

Equipment

Soft toothbrush/fluoride toothpaste/water/ disposable cup/receiver such as a disposable kidney bowl/foam sticks/towel tissues/lip balm/disposable gloves and apron/suction machine

Procedure

1. Explain procedure and gain consent.
2. Wash hands, put on protective clothing.
3. Roll patient onto their side and position yourself directly in front of them.
4. Position towel around the neck and chest area.
5. As rinsing maybe difficult, squeeze less than recommended amount of toothpaste on the brush (DOH 2014) and wet the brush with some water poured into the disposable cup.
6. Hold brush at a 45° angle to the teeth and brush using circular motion clean the gums and outer surfaces of the teeth and then the inner surfaces of the teeth. Holding the brush at 90° clean the biting surfaces using the same circular movement of the brush and then the tongue.
7. Use sponge foam sticks rinse. Wet a stick in a little water, applying (twisting movement) in the mouth to absorb the toothpaste and any debris, remove and dispose. Repeat (with a clean foam stick each time) until all toothpaste and debris is removed. If required, suction out excessive water using a yanker sucker. Care needs to be taken when giving mouth care to the unconscious patient or a patient with swallowing problems because of the risk of choking. ASSESS AIRWAY AT ALL TIMES DURING THE PROCEDURE.
8. Apply lip balm/yellow soft paraffin sparingly to the lips.
9. Rinse out toothbrush under running water and store in a clean disposable cup on the patient's locker to dry.
10. Dispose of apron/gloves in clinical waste and wash your hands.
11. Documentation.

Mouth (Oral Cavity)

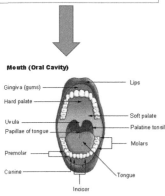

Gingiva (gums)
Hard palate
Uvula
Papillae of tongue
Premolar
Canine
Incisor
Lips
Soft palate
Palatine tonsil
Molars
Tongue

Procedure for shaving

1. Explain procedure and gain consent.
2. Use either patient's own razor or a disposable razor.
3. Wash hands before and after.
4. Moisten patient's face with a warm wet washcloth, apply soap/shaving lotion on patient's face.
5. Shave gently, following direction of the hair, being careful of skin creases near mouth and nose. Shave in short strokes while carefully stretching the skin flat with your free hand.
6. Rinse the patient's face thoroughly with warm water and disposable wipe.
7. Dispose of razors in sharps bin.

FIGURE 4.7 Oral care and shaving

PSYCHOSOCIAL

Non-verbal communication will not be experienced by the person who is unconscious but will be by their visiting family and friends or those with impaired consciousness.

- **No use of words**: no words but use of gestures, facial expressions, eye contact, physical proximity, touching.
- **Culturally determined**: learnt in childhood, passed on by parents and others. Adoption of mannerisms of one's cultural group.
- **Different meaning**: non-verbal symbols can have many meanings. Cross-culture aspects give various meanings to same expression in respect of non-verbal communication.
- **Vague and imprecise**: Since in this communication there is no use of words or language which expresses clear meaning.
- **May conflict with verbal message**: non-verbal communication is so deeply rooted, so unconscious, that you can express a verbal message and then directly contradict it with a non-verbal message.
- **Largely unconscious**: non-verbal communication is unconscious in the sense that it is usually not planned nor rehearsed. It comes almost instantaneously.
- **Shows feelings and attitudes**: through facial expressions, gestures, body movements, use of eyes.
- **Informality**: non-verbal communication does not follow any rules, formality or structure like other communication. Most of the cases people unconsciously and habitually engaged in non-verbal communication by moving the various parts of the body.

Communication also conveys a sense of being respected, valued, and safe.

- Adapt your communication style to communicate better with others, particularly when the patient is unconscious.
- Learn about the cultural etiquette of the patient and adapt appropriately.
- **How** things are said are important. Tone of voice is vital to convey positive emotion. Be aware of betraying, through the tone of voice, feelings and opinions that may intimidate or belittle the patient.
- With different levels of consciousness, be astute in reading and interpreting non-verbal behaviours and gestures. Gestures and body language vary and are an intricate aspect in communication.
- Ask questions of relatives/friends for clarification of norms and practices, for example, unwritten rules from other cultures.
- Accommodate language barriers where possible. The use of relatives may need to be used when talking to the unconscious patient (explaining simple tasks etc.) who speaks very little or no English.
- Use inclusive language – since diversity includes gender, reframe from the use of male dominant language, i.e. men, he, him.
- Suspend judgmental tendency to evaluate statements and actions of other persons. Try to comprehend feelings and thoughts that are behind the expression.
- Although verbal communication with an unconscious patient is a one-sided experience, nurses need to be perceptive of the patient's nonverbal signs. Recognise high anxiety is common in cross-cultural experiences. This will be displayed non verbally (e.g. increased heart rate, blood pressure, breathing rate).

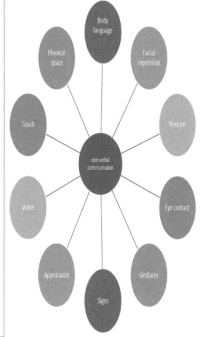

FIGURE 4.8 Psychosocial needs

Activity: now test yourself

1. List the five main priorities in caring for an unconscious patient.

2. Why is the unconscious state potentially life-threatening?

3. **True** or **false**? During the breakdown of protein, nitrogen is lost from the body. When nitrogen exceeds supply a catabolic situation for the body is created. This can result in muscle breakdown and, in severe cases, breakdown of intercostal muscles.

4. Why is it important to address the psychosocial needs of the patient, particularly verbal communication and therapeutic use of touch?

Answers

1. The five priorities are: a) maintaining a clear airway; b) assessing and monitoring level of consciousness; c) assessing and monitoring vital signs; d) assessing and maintaining hydration and nutrition needs; e) appropriate nursing intervention/care management.

2. Loss of gag reflex – compromised coughing and swallowing which means that the airway can become blocked very easily leading to asphyxiation. Aspiration can also occur.

3. True.

4. Hearing is the last sense to go and the first to return. Patients should be spoken to gently before being touched.

Reflection: ask yourself

1. What do I know now that I didn't know before?

2. What am I confused/unclear about?

3. What areas do I need to focus on?

4. My action plan for further learning (make objectives SMART – Specific/Measurable/Achievable/Realistic/Time-bound):

CHAPTER 5

Pain

Sheila Cunningham

Overview

Assessing and managing pain are essential components of nursing practice. Pain is referred to as a complex concept in all aspects of life: it can be physical, psychological and social and is uniquely subjective. Nurses will encounter patients with pain across all clinical settings and age ranges (RCN, 2015) and thus assessing and managing it effectively are fundamental care skills to acquire.

Link to *Future Nurse Proficiencies* (NMC 2018)

Annexe B: Nursing procedures, Sections 3 and 10. Specifically, 3.1: observe and assess comfort and pain levels and rest and sleep patterns; 3.5: take appropriate action to reduce or minimise pain or discomfort; and 10.1: observe and assess the need for intervention for people, families and carers, identify, assess and respond appropriately to uncontrolled symptoms and signs of distress including pain, nausea, thirst, constipation, restlessness, agitation, anxiety and depression.

Expected knowledge

- Sensory pathways and nerve conduction
- Sources of pain and situations where it may be experienced (planned and unplanned)
- Your own experience of pain and its biopsychosocial impacts.

Introduction

Everyone in their lifetime will experience pain at various times to varying degrees. Pain can be useful as an indicator that something is not right or a condition is occurring; it can also be useful as a protective mechanism in injury to avoid deterioration. However, there are also times when pain serves no useful purpose and continues long after the injury, healing or repair is over. Pain is a common feature shared by everyone at whatever age; however, the experience of and meaning attributed to pain is unique to individuals, commanding an individualised approach to assessment and management. Pain can be organic, related to tissue damage or changes, or it could be an emotional experience or loss – but whatever the cause or nature of pain, it is essential to accept the individual's interpretation and description or reaction to it and tailor care accordingly.

The widespread prevalence of pain reinforces the need for all health care professionals to be equipped with comprehensive pain knowledge and education. However, not all health care professionals require the same type or level of pain-related knowledge and skills. Pain is often poorly managed and has impacts on not only the person experiencing pain but also their family and friends and the wider sphere of socio-economic costs. Pain affects all populations globally. A pain audit in the UK reported that each year over five million people in the United Kingdom develop pain, specifically chronic pain, but only two-thirds will recover (Price et al., 2012). Furthermore, an estimated 11% of adults and 8% of children suffer severe pain, which accounts for a huge proportion of the population (7.8 million) in the UK. It was also identified that there are some significant predictors of chronic pain in the community, i.e. advanced age, being female and socio-economic status aspects such as housing and type of employment. Whilst this study is a little dated, the situation is unlikely to have changed much and indicates that this is an ongoing problem that requires adequate nursing knowledge and skills preparation. Such information as this aids assessment and management.

Content

Pain sensations	Causes of pain	Pain types
Consequences of unrelieved pain	Pain experience	Pain management

Learning outcomes

- Outline the pain mechanisms and classification of pain types
- Identify methods to assess pain and determine effect of interventions
- Describe pharmacological and non-pharmacological approaches to pain relief
- Identify the skills needed to manage pain
- Reflect on your knowledge of pain physiology, causes and impact on patients' lives and wellbeing and effective nursing interventions to relieve pain.

Key background

Every nurse should be able to assess and manage pain effectively. Nurses are central to patient care and due to the close and frequent contact in a variety of settings such as hospital wards or clinics, homecare settings, residential settings or the community they play a critical role in effective pain assessment and management. This places the nurse in a unique position to:

- Identify patients who may be experiencing pain
- Assess patients in pain for cause, duration, location and effect, which may include the patient's family and significant others
- Plan and initiate interventions to manage the pain
- Evaluate the effectiveness of those interventions.

Given nurses' position in patient care they need to be knowledgeable about pain mechanisms, the epidemiology of pain and barriers to effective pain control. Fundamentally this is core to adequate assessment and also management. They also ought to be aware of frequently encountered pain conditions, variables which influence the patient's perception of and response to pain. This further extends to the awareness and appropriate use of valid and reliable methods of clinical pain assessment and a range of available methods for relieving pain. The goals of pain management are to a large extent determined by those experiencing pain themselves.

Pain is viewed as a biopsychosocial phenomenon that includes social, psychological and biological factors. It has been reported over many decades to be a multidimensional and complex phenomenon that requires comprehensive, ongoing assessment and effective management. Since it is multidimensional, this necessitates an interprofessional approach to assessment and management to be effective, which can be coordinated by the nurse providing care. All professionals serve as advocates for the person in pain and adopt practice which ensures that pain treatment is based on ethical principles and evidence-based guidelines.

Who has pain?

In 2017, 34% of all adults had chronic pain.
- Varied with age: 16% among adults aged 16 to 24 years, and 53% among adults aged 75 and over.
- Highest amongst those with lower incomes.
                                    (HSE, 2019)

Consequences include:
- a lower quality of life,
- impacts on mental health,
- job losses, and
- limiting daily activities.

Chronic pain in HSE is defined as 'pain or discomfort that had troubled the participant all of the time, or on and off, for more than the last three months'.   (HSE, 2019)

Physical and emotional pain?
- Research points to a 'shared network' and patterns brain processing of pain experiences. Both realities (physical and emotional) pain connect. (Bruneau et al., 2012)
- Termed: somatomotor-somatosensory networks and emotional-interceptive networks.

Terms used to describe pain by patients:
- Aching
- Cramping
- Fearful
- Gnawing/heavy
- Hot or burning
- Sharp/shooting
- Sickening
- Splitting/stabbing
- Punishing or cruel
- Tender/throbbing
- Tiring or exhausting

PAIN – WHAT IS IT?

Defining pain
An aversive sensory and emotional experience typically caused by, or resembling that caused by, actual or potential tissue injury. (ISAP, 2019)

- Pain is always a subjective experience that is influenced to varying degrees by biological, psychological, and social factors.
- Pain and nociception are different phenomena: the experience of pain cannot be reduced to activity in sensory pathways.
- Through their life experiences, individuals learn the concept of pain and its applications.
- A person's report of an experience as pain should be accepted as such and respected.
- Although pain usually serves an adaptive role, it may have adverse effects on function and social and psychological well-being.
- Verbal description is only one of several behaviours to express pain; inability to communicate does not negate the possibility that a human or a non-human animal experiences pain.
                                    (IASP, 2019)

Physical and behavioural responses to pain

Physical/physiology:
- Signs of stress: sweating, anxiety, restlessness.
- Increased heart and respiratory rate and blood pressure.
- Nausea or vomiting (gastric stasis).

Behavioural:
- Withdrawal not engaging and being quiet.
- Aggression or anger and verbal abuse.
- Facial expressions: grimace, frowning, moaning, howling.
- Pacing, rubbing affected area.
- Crying, screaming.
- Young children or other non verbal people: may exhibit altered behaviour or refusal to eat or be withdrawn.
- Other groups: those confused, with cognitive impairment or unconscious – all experience pain – behaviours may change but ought be observed for.

Influences on pain perceptions:
- Influenced by appraisal and past experiences.
- Responses are modified by culture and social experiences. Children learn acceptable behaviours to use during pain episode.
- Some societies take a 'stoic' approach to pain.
- Expression of pain varies (socially, culturally) and with age.

FIGURE 5.1 Pain: what is it?

TYPES AND CHARACTERISTICS OF PAIN

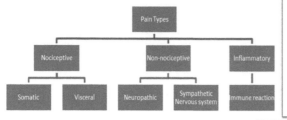

Classification of pain

Pain may be classified according to factors such as
- Origin/pathology
- Timescale (acute or chronic – *very indistinct*)
- Whether nociceptive or neuropathic

These are broad distinctions however do guide assessment influence pain management approaches.

Nociceptive pain
- Represents the normal response to noxious insult or injury of tissues such as skin, muscles, visceral organs, joints, tendons, or bones.
- It arises from the stimulation of specific pain receptors. These receptors can respond to heat, cold, vibration, stretch and chemical stimuli released from damaged cells. Examples include:
- Somatic: tissues such as skin, muscle, joints, bones, and ligaments
- Visceral: internal organs of the main body cavities and smooth muscle; may feel like a vague deep ache, sometimes being cramping or colicky in nature. Often described by patients as 'referred' meaning the pain sensation produces referred pain distant to the site; pelvic pain referring pain to the lower back.

PAIN

Acute Pain
- Brief duration.
- Sudden onset (mild to severe).
- Range of intensity.
- Frequently encountered in all care settings.
- Akin to nociceptive pain – linked to tissue damage (somatic or visceral).
- Time limited – eases with healing/repair.
- May be predictable e.g. Sickle cell crisis episodes, or surgery.
- Triggers primitive survival instincts (fight/flight) and the features of that.
- Readily treated with analgesia (drugs).
- Caution needed when assessing this and physiological effects in people with memory issues, pre-verbal children, or communication difficulties.

Non-nociceptive pain
or **Neuropathic pain**: caused by a primary lesion or disease in the somatosensory nervous system.
- Nerve Degeneration – multiple sclerosis, stroke, brain haemorrhage, oxygen starvation
- Nerve Pressure – trapped nerve
- Nerve Inflammation – torn or slipped vertebral disc
- Nerve Infection – shingles and other viral infections

Examples include, but are not limited to, diabetic neuropathy, spinal cord injury pain, phantom limb (post-amputation) pain, and post-stroke central pain.

Inflammatory pain
Activation and sensitization of the nociceptive pain pathway by a variety of chemicals released at a site of tissue inflammation.

Examples include appendicitis, rheumatoid arthritis, inflammatory bowel disease, and herpes zoster (shingles).

FIGURE 5.2 Types and characteristics of pain

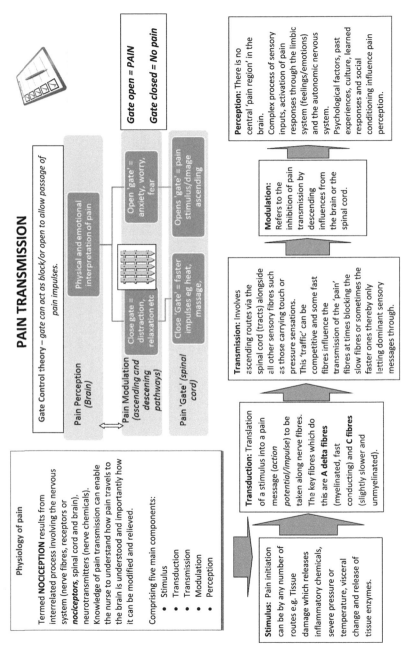

FIGURE 5.3 Pain transmission

PAIN LANGUAGE

Communicating pain: The language of pain description enables communication of assessment and interventions to colleagues and aids multidisciplinary care.

Term	Explanation
Allodynia	Pain due to a stimulus that does not normally provoke pain for example heightened sensitivity following burn.
Hyperalgesia	Increased pain from a stimulus that normally provokes pain.
Neuralgia	Pain in the distribution of a nerve or nerves.
Neuritis	Inflammation of a nerve or nerves.
Nociception	The neural process of receiving and interpreting a sensation as a noxious stimuli.
Pain threshold	The minimum intensity of a stimulus that is perceived as painful.
Pain tolerance level	The maximum intensity of a pain-producing stimulus that a person is willing to accept in a given situation.
Time course of pain:	Acute pain: pain of less than 3 to 6 months duration Chronic pain: pain lasting for more than 3-6 months, or persisting beyond the course of an acute disease, or after tissue healing is complete. Acute-on-chronic pain: acute pain episode on top of underlying chronic pain.

Verbal challenges

Some groups of patients may have difficulties expressing pain:
- language barriers,
- children,
- elderly,
- those with cognitive impairment,
- learning disabilities or mental health problems.

Requires skilled nursing communication and observation remembering the total pain experience.

COMMON MYTHS

Pain is a natural side effect of aging.	Sometimes it can be or from physical wear and tear is normal. Differs from chronic pain.
Ignore pain, it will go away.	Can have serious consequences, self-medication might mask features and underlying cause.
Exercise makes pain worse.	Depends on the cause of the pain. If it is not traumatic then exercise such can be key to pain control or rehabilitation.
Painkillers are addictive if taken long term.	The risk of addiction is exaggerated however if analgesia is needed it ought be taken.
Chronic pain can kill you.	It can have a profound effect on quality of life. Certain severe situations may prompt suicidal feelings if pain seems unbearable. Psychological support is essential.
Dwelling on pain will make it worse.	Dwelling on the pain can emphasize it and distraction or other approaches can make it feel less intrusive.

Suggestion for communicating with patients in pain

- Be open and honest tell them - you are there do your best to relieve their pain.
- Remain calm and show empathy.
- Express concerns for the patient's feelings and emotions.
- Use patient-centred interviewing and caring communication skills in daily practice.
- Use age appropriate language or patients own 'pain language'
- Encourage patients to write down their questions in preparation for appointments or episodes of care.
- Allow time - it improves patient-centred interviewing, shared decision-making, and improved patient-carer communication in pain assessment and management.

FIGURE 5.4 Pain language

ASSESSMENT OF PAIN

Why assess?

Accurate assessment is a key rationale in the process of pain management.

- The aim is to identify factors (physical and non-physical) which affect patient's perception of pain to then select the most appropriate management approach.
- Assessment is a challenge because it is subjective and multidimensional.
- *Locus of control*: may account for individual differences – levels of control and dependence.
- Gender differences – socialisation and levels of expression of pain experience.
- Culture: linked to belief systems and social behaviours and levels of expression or meaning of pain.

Pain assessment tools

There are number of validated subjective tools examples include :

- *Visual Analogue Scale* (VAS): for acute and chronic pain. Scores are recorded by making a handwritten mark on a 10-cm line that represents a continuum between "no pain" and "worst pain."

No pain--Worst pain

- *Verbal Numerical Rating Scale* (VNRS): similar to the VAS above, however on this scale 0 represents 'no pain' and 10 'worst pain imaginable'.
- *McGill Pain Questionnaire*: consists of groupings of words that describe and locate pain e.g. tugging, sharp and nagging. Once the patient has selected their pain words, the nurse assigns a numerical score, called the Pain Rating Index.
- *Abbey Pain Scale*: an observational pain tool for people with dementia who cannot verbalise – completed by the nurse or observer.
- *Wong-Baker faces pain scale* – a series of faces ranging from a happy face at 0, or "no hurt", to a crying face at 10, which represents "hurts like the worst pain imaginable"

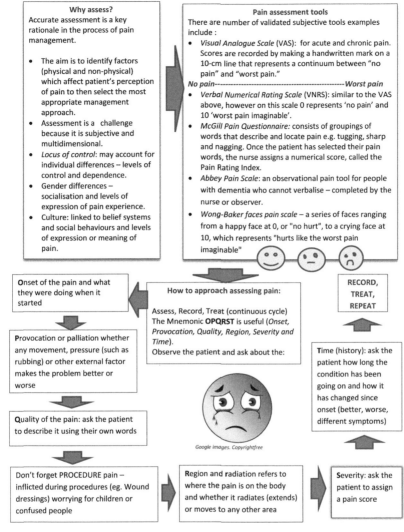

Onset of the pain and what they were doing when it started

Provocation or palliation whether any movement, pressure (such as rubbing) or other external factor makes the problem better or worse

Quality of the pain: ask the patient to describe it using their own words

Don't forget PROCEDURE pain – inflicted during procedures (eg. Wound dressings) worrying for children or confused people

How to approach assessing pain:

Assess, Record, Treat (continuous cycle)
The Mnemonic **OPQRST** is useful (*Onset, Provocation, Quality, Region, Severity and Time*).
Observe the patient and ask about the:

Google images. Copyrightfree

Region and radiation refers to where the pain is on the body and whether it radiates (extends) or moves to any other area

RECORD, TREAT, REPEAT

Time (history): ask the patient how long the condition has been going on and how it has changed since onset (better, worse, different symptoms)

Severity: ask the patient to assign a pain score

FIGURE 5.5 Assessment of pain

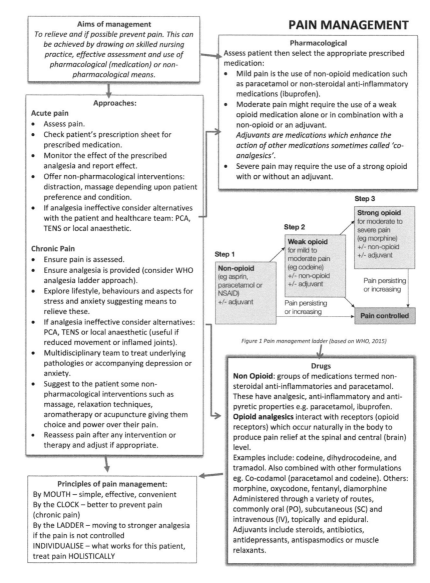

Aims of management
To relieve and if possible prevent pain. This can be achieved by drawing on skilled nursing practice, effective assessment and use of pharmacological (medication) or non-pharmacological means.

PAIN MANAGEMENT

Pharmacological
Assess patient then select the appropriate prescribed medication:
- Mild pain is the use of non-opioid medication such as paracetamol or non-steroidal anti-inflammatory medications (ibuprofen).
- Moderate pain might require the use of a weak opioid medication alone or in combination with a non-opioid or an adjuvant.
 Adjuvants are medications which enhance the action of other medications sometimes called 'co-analgesics'.
- Severe pain may require the use of a strong opioid with or without an adjuvant.

Approaches:
Acute pain
- Assess pain.
- Check patient's prescription sheet for prescribed medication.
- Monitor the effect of the prescribed analgesia and report effect.
- Offer non-pharmacological interventions: distraction, massage depending upon patient preference and condition.
- If analgesia ineffective consider alternatives with the patient and healthcare team: PCA, TENS or local anaesthetic.

Chronic Pain
- Ensure pain is assessed.
- Ensure analgesia is provided (consider WHO analgesia ladder approach).
- Explore lifestyle, behaviours and aspects for stress and anxiety suggesting means to relieve these.
- If analgesia ineffective consider alternatives: PCA, TENS or local anaesthetic (useful if reduced movement or inflamed joints).
- Multidisciplinary team to treat underlying pathologies or accompanying depression or anxiety.
- Suggest to the patient some non-pharmacological interventions such as massage, relaxation techniques, aromatherapy or acupuncture giving them choice and power over their pain.
- Reassess pain after any intervention or therapy and adjust if appropriate.

Step 1
Non-opioid
(eg asprin, paracetamol or NSAID)
+/- adjuvant

Pain persisting or increasing

Step 2
Weak opioid
for mild to moderate pain
(eg codeine)
+/- non-opioid
+/- adjuvant

Pain persisting or increasing

Step 3
Strong opioid
for moderate to severe pain
(eg morphine)
+/- non-opioid
+/- adjuvant

Pain persisting or increasing

Pain controlled

Figure 1 Pain management ladder (based on WHO, 2015)

Drugs
Non Opioid: groups of medications termed non-steroidal anti-inflammatories and paracetamol. These have analgesic, anti-inflammatory and anti-pyretic properties e.g. paracetamol, ibuprofen.
Opioid analgesics interact with receptors (opioid receptors) which occur naturally in the body to produce pain relief at the spinal and central (brain) level.
Examples include: codeine, dihydrocodeine, and tramadol. Also combined with other formulations eg. Co-codamol (paracetamol and codeine). Others: morphine, oxycodone, fentanyl, diamorphine
Administered through a variety of routes, commonly oral (PO), subcutaneous (SC) and intravenous (IV), topically and epidural.
Adjuvants include steroids, antibiotics, antidepressants, antispasmodics or muscle relaxants.

Principles of pain management:
By MOUTH – simple, effective, convenient
By the CLOCK – better to prevent pain (chronic pain)
By the LADDER – moving to stronger analgesia if the pain is not controlled
INDIVIDUALISE – what works for this patient, treat pain HOLISTICALLY

FIGURE 5.6 Pain management

Patient Controlled Analgesia (PCA)

Analgesia (often morphine or diamorphine) is infused using an infusion pump and timing device and is self-controlled by the patient so adequate amounts of analgesia can be self-administered 'on demand'. Routes for PCA include subcutaneous, intravenous (IV – the most common) and epidural. Monitoring for levels of sedation are needed with this form of analgesia administration.

OTHER PAIN RELIEF APPROACHES

Non-pharmacological methods of pain relief

Emotional and psychological interventions:
Information/education and building trust
- Breathing exercises
- Visual imagery
- Cognitive behavioural therapy (CBT)
- Yoga/tai chi
- Art/music relaxation
- Distraction (guided imagery)
- Relaxation or meditation
- Spiritual or reflective activities related to the patient's belief system

Physical interventions:
- Heat or cold therapy
- Exercise or Rest
- Body position/movements
- Massage

Care of a patient with PCA
- Explain procedure, gain patient consent, maintain hand hygiene.
- Check the prescription of the PCA and the equipment: patient label on syringe, drug dose, concentration, date and time. Note how much is left in the syringe.
- Check the PCA programme (loading dose, lock-out duration, basal rate of infusion, and bolus dose (patient demand dose).
- Record the history from the PCA device (requests for doses and how much given) to inform pain level and efficacy of pain relief.
- Check the IV site for signs of redness, swelling or discomfort.
- Check the IV line is functioning and correctly labelled for date/time of line change.
- Assess the patient for pain and determine the level of pain relief.
- Observe for alterations in pulse or blood pressure or respiration rate and any altered consciousness. (Note Opioids cause respiratory depression) If any observed report immediately.
- Document the findings reporting any concerns.

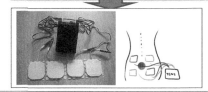

Trans Cutaneous Nerve Stimulation (TENS)

Patient/parents can set this up themselves – guidance is:
1. Ensure the machine is switched off before starting. Then insert battery (instruction booklet).
2. Plug the attaching leads into the electrode pads then into the machine at the lead connector.
3. Make sure that the area of skin where the electrode pads will be placed is clean and dry.
4. Remove the electrodes from the plastic sheet.
5. Apply the electrode pads to the areas of pain (at least 2–3 cm apart) and not be touching.
6. Gently switch on the TENS machine, the green LED light will indicate that the machine is switched on. Ask patient/child to turn up the dial slowly until the sensation through the electrode pads is strong but comfortable.
7. The patient/child should feel a gentle tingle or buzzing sensation in the area of pain. If it is not in the right place, switch off the machine and re-positioning the electrode pads.
8. If uncomfortable or allergic then switch off, remove and report to nurse or doctor.

Complementary/alternative interventions:
- Acupuncture/ Acupressure
- Biofield therapies – which include Reiki, therapeutic touch, and healing touch
- Reflexology
- Electrostimulation (TENS)
- Herbs (topical capsaicin)

FIGURE 5.7 Other pain relief approaches

Activity: now test yourself

1. Which four processes are involved in acute nociceptive pain?

    a) transudation, transmission, modulation and perception

    b) translocation, transmission, modulation and perception

    c) translocation, perception, modulation and threshold

    d) transduction, transmission, modulation and perception.

2. Which of the following statements about pain threshold is **true**?

    a) It is the lowest intensity at which an experience of pain is sensed.

    b) It is the greatest level of pain which the person is prepared to tolerate.

    c) It varies widely among cultures and ethnicities.

    d) It is influenced by previous pain experiences.

3. Which of the following statements is **true**?

    a) Paracetamol is a mild opioid.

    b) The WHO analgesic ladder refers to giving more of every pain medication together to ease pain.

    c) Morphine is used for any type of pain from mild to moderate.

    d) Ibuprofen has a nonsteroidal anti-inflammatory action and thus relieves pain this way.

4. What key principles are there when assessing pain?

    a) Record physical features such as pulse and blood pressure and facial expressions to determine level of pain.

    b) Review patient's medication usage if they are taking more analgesics than they are in pain.

c) Use process such as *OPQRST* (Onset, Provocation, Quality, Region, Severity and Time).

d) Observe the patient whilst they are not aware and see if they look like they are in pain using the *SBAR* approach (Situation, Background, Assessment, Recommendation).

5. Patient-controlled analgesia (PCA) refers to which of the following?

a) medication which is deemed not dangerous and patients can take themselves

b) medication which is given post-surgery by nurses because patients are unable to take it themselves

c) when patients have a choice of what medication to take for painful periods

d) medication which can be given intravenously and where the bolus doses are controlled by patients themselves.

6. Which of the following are non-pharmacological approaches to managing pain (tick all that apply)?

a) transcutaneous nerve stimulation (TENS)

b) aromatherapy

c) guided imagery

d) breathing exercises

e) hot or cold therapy

f) acupuncture

g) shiatsu

h) vitamins.

Answers

1. d) *Acute nociceptive pain involves the four processes of transduction, transmission, modulation and perception. 'Transudation' is the movement of a fluid through a membrane. 'Translocation' is the transfer of a chromosomal segment to a different site on the same chromosome or to another chromosome.*

2. a) *The threshold refers to the lowest level at which a stimulus is transmitted to be perceived as a sensation, in this instance 'pain'. It is not correct to view the greatest amount of pain experienced as a threshold; that may be an issue of tolerance but is not acceptable in any care situation. Whilst former experiences and culture can affect expression of pain, this is not exactly the same as threshold.*

3. d) *Ibuprofen is categorised as a nonsteroidal anti-inflammatory drug (NSAID) which works by blocking an enzyme pathway that makes prostaglandin which causes inflammation and pain. NSAIDS are useful for pain caused by infections or inflammations and also have antipyretic action (reducing fever).*

   Morphine is an opioid and is used for severe pain as it has strong effects and side effects whilst paracetamol is not an opioid and is used for mild to moderate pain. The WHO analgesic ladder is a pathway to assessment and an increase in the 'type' of medication, not adding but substituting – if adding this might be dangerous and lead to toxicity.

4. c) *Watching or observing patients and not asking them about pain means that nurses make a judgement which is flawed as pain is expressed and felt in different ways. The correct response is c), since this approach focuses clearly on pain – onset, provocation, quality, region, severity and time. The acronym SBAR is a communication tool which could be used to communicate the findings after using the OPQRS tool.*

5. d) *Patient-controlled analgesia means it is under the patient's control – not the type of medication but certainly the number of doses. This is set up to 'lock out' so they cannot overdose but gives them the control especially post-surgery, and both features (medication and control) contribute to a tailored, more positive pain management experience.*

6. Options a)–g) are all correct; h) is not. *There are a wide range of non-pharmacological approaches to pain relief – some are referred to as physical approaches and some as complementary or alternative therapies. There is no documented evidence of vitamins having any effect on pain; however, optimal physical support and replacement is of benefit to general healing if not pain control specifically.*

Reflection: ask yourself

1. What do I know now that I didn't know before?

2. What am I confused/unclear about?

3. What areas do I need to focus on?

4. My action plan for further learning (make objectives SMART – Specific/Measurable/Achievable/Realistic/Time-bound):

CHAPTER 6

Sleep

Sheila Cunningham

Overview

Sleep is a fundamental need and yet the purpose of it remains unclear. Knowledge about sleep and sleep disorders is important for health care professionals since it affects individuals as well as the wider family and communities within which individuals live. Like in many activities of daily living, nurses and health care professionals caring for patients are in a central position to evaluate and intervene to promote sleep for patients or clients. Nurses are also not immune. Shift pattern stresses and busy lives mean nurses need to manage their own health risks and optimise their health and wellbeing. Part of this includes a more comprehensive understanding of sleep and circadian and other rhythms as well as minimising the impacts of sleep deprivation.

Link to *Future Nurse Proficiencies* (NMC 2018)

Platform 4 Providing and evaluating care. Specifically, 4.1: demonstrate and apply an understanding of what is important to people and how to use this knowledge to ensure their needs for safety, dignity, privacy, comfort and sleep can be met.

Annexe B, Part 2: Specifically, 3.1: observe and assess comfort and pain levels and rest and sleep patterns and 3.6: take appropriate action to reduce fatigue, minimise insomnia and support improved rest and sleep hygiene.

Expected knowledge

- Fundamental process of life (basic life functions) as related to activities of daily living
- Comfort measures and physical and psychological signs of comfort and relaxation.

Introduction

The need to educate the future nursing workforce to increase understanding of healthy sleep practices, adverse health consequences of impaired sleep and common sleep disorders is pressing. This is reinforced in the professional competencies for nursing students moving forward into the 21st century. Sleep therefore is becoming a more established part of the undergraduate nursing curriculum. In addition, increased exposure of this topic in literature and media will reinforce understanding and skills around this essential but ill-defined phenomenon.

Content

Physiology of sleep	Purpose and function of sleep	Promoting sleep
Sleep disorders	Wakefulness and biorhythms	Factors disrupting sleep

Learning outcomes

- Discuss the purpose of sleep and issues with sleep deprivation
- Outline the mechanism of sleep and the features of each stage in the sleep cycle
- Explain factors which impair or promote sleep and change over a lifespan
- Discuss sleep environments and what is meant by 'sleep hygiene'
- Reflect on your own personal experiences of sleep including changes over your own lifespan and with shift work and professional functioning.

Key background

Sleep is important for healing and recovery. Patients in hospitals are subject to noise and care practices which result too often in sleep deprivation and as such it is a major concern for hospital staff. This is not unique to hospitals and also extends to other care environments linked to a variety of factors. Several causes of sleep disturbance have been identified, including patients' anxiety about their care and condition; pain; and environmental factors, such as noise, light and the administration of nursing care (Patel et al., 2008; Pilkington, 2013). As mentioned noise is a factor which is frequently cited as a major contributor to sleep disruption especially in hospitals. Fragmented sleep in hospital inpatients may also be exacerbated by light at night, but also by relatively low light levels by day; these may be insufficient to maintain a normal circadian rhythm with adequate differentiation between day and night (Bernhofer et al., 2014). Night-time nursing activities are also recognised as a major contributor to sleep disruption in hospitals and the seemingly apparent obliviousness of nurses to noise levels and sources complicates this (Norton et al., 2015).

During sleep, a situation of non-responsiveness to sensory stimuli from the environment occurs. As such it points to sleep being potentially supported through three basic mechanisms:

- reduction in stimuli
- interruption of the transmission of sensory stimuli from the environment; or
- reducing the brain's attention to the stimuli.

It has been documented (Pisani et al., 2015) that if poor sleep develops in a hospital setting as a consequence of an acute illness, it can persist for an extended period of time after discharge. It is also one of the most frequently cited stressful experiences for patients who have been critically ill (Pisani et al., 2015). For those afflicted, assessment of sleep may be undertaken. This includes techniques such as polysomnography, a technique that records bio-physiological changes and provides the most accurate and detailed information about the processes and physical impacts of sleep.

In reference to reducing stimuli of noise and light, earplugs and eye masks offer an easy and affordable solution for improving sleep. Five studies evaluating the impact of earplugs and eye masks in isolation were reviewed pointing to some strong positive solutions. In one study patients with earplugs reported significant improvements in sleep depth, ease of falling asleep, satisfaction, amount, movement during sleep and waking in the night (Norton et al., 2015).

Older people are prone to multiple pathologies and these disease processes may impact on and also obscure their need for effective sleep and rest. There are a few concepts which relate to the process and need for sleep, namely sleep architecture and sleep hygiene. 'Sleep architecture' is a term that refers to the mechanics of sleep or sleep stages. 'Sleep hygiene' refers to measures or interventions used to promote sleep and a person-centred approach is necessary, with support from specialist agencies to achieve effective sleep hygiene. Any of these are considerations for assessment but also solutions to sleep concerns. The duration and quality of sleep alters throughout life and it appears that with advancing ages the need for long periods of sleep may diminish. However, the quality of the sleep experiences, i.e. feeling rested and refreshed, should be the same (Bephage, 2005). There are additional challenges to recognising, diagnosing and treating sleep disorders in older adults with dementia and those in long-term care facilities. Needless to say these further complicate the clinical management of sleep disorders in these patients or clients (Lavoie et al., 2018).

Normal lifespan changes may also impact on sleep. A substantial number of women experience sleep difficulties in the approach to menopause and beyond. It is reported that up to 26% of women experience severe symptoms that impact daytime functioning (Baker et al., 2018). This is most likely associated with fluctuating hormone levels and the emergence of physiological and psychological symptoms such as hot flushes (vasomotor effects) and mood changes resulting in sleep disturbances.

In a relatively recent systematic review Bartel and Gradisar (2016) concluded that longitudinally there are consistent links between young people's use of technology and sleep. The use of technology in a variety of settings for study or leisure including the use of social media often means that a considerable proportion of the day is spent on such devices. Although the literature points to a link between technology use and sleep disturbance among adolescents and young people it is unclear if this is caus-ing sleep problems or if technology is an activity responding to problems with sleep. In any event sleep issues require a holistic approach at any age and for any cause(s).

Nurses have a professional responsibility to safely support patient recovery and this means attending to rest and sleep as part of nursing care. They also ought to be in a position to take decisions and appropriate action to reduce fatigue, minimise insomnia and support improved rest and sleep hygiene in their patients. As humans who need to function it is essential nurses also reflect on their own practices (sleep hygiene, etc.) within themselves for optimal professional performance.

WAKEFULNESS AND SLEEP

Sleep-wake cycles

Sleep, rest and relaxation are necessary for wellbeing and health maintenance. Comprises a fundamental need on the Maslow hierarchy.

Biorhythms – cyclical patterns of biological functions unique to individuals. Examples include: sleep-wake, fluctuations in body temperature, alterations in hormones release, heart rate and mood.

A **circadian rhythm** (or *diurnal rhythm*) is a natural, internal process of physical, mental, and behavioral changes that regulates the sleep-wake cycle and repeats roughly every 24 hours. *Varies across the lifespan.*

- These can influence hormone release, eating habits and digestion, body temperature, and other important bodily functions.
- Irregular rhythms have been linked to various chronic health conditions, such as sleep disorders, obesity, diabetes, depression, bipolar disorder, and seasonal affective disorder.
- They respond primarily to light and darkness detected by photoreceptors in an organism's *Suprachiasmatic nucleus* (SCN) in brain.
- The study of circadian rhythms is referred to as *chronobiology*.

SLEEP?

Sleep is defined as a state of partial unconsciousness from which person is aroused by stimulation (Marieb, 2018).

Sleep is a naturally recurring state of mind and body, characterized by decreased ability to react to stimuli and surroundings.

- It is distinguished from wakefulness.
- It is more reactive than a coma or disorders of consciousness.

During sleep:
- Arterial blood pressure, heart rate and respiratory decrease.
- Metabolism is reduced.
- Skeletal activity reduces.
- Growth hormone secretion increases.
- Learning, memory and reasoning occur.
- Concentration improves in waking hours.

Neurotransmitters associated with sleep INDUCING/REDUCING

- 5-hydroxytryptamine (5-HT) (Serotonin)
- Norepinephrine
- Acetylcholine
- Orexin/Hypocretin
- Dopamine
- Gamma-amino butyric acid (GABA)
- Glutamate
- Adenosine
- Cortisol
- Melatonin
- Growth hormone releasing hormone (GHRH)

Reticular Formation (RF) Brain Role:

RF consists of more than 100 small neural networks (thalamus, cerebral cortex, hypothalamus etc.), with varied functions including:
- Control motor activity
- Pain modulation (transmission)
- Filters sensory inputs (habituation)
- Sleep/wake periods: (*Reticular activating system*)
  1. High activity = stimulated and awake
  2. Low activity = relax and fall asleep
- ACTION through neurotransmitters (eg. Dopamine, serotonin etc).

FIGURE 6.1 Wakefulness and sleep

PHYSIOLOGY OF SLEEP

Function of sleep

Not entirely clear. Thought be beneficial for:

- Consolidation of learning and experiences.
- Expressions of concerns or sub consciousness.
- Growth and tissue repair processes.
- Immune health – evidenced through fluctuation of Interleukin-1 (white blood cell signalling protein) parallel with sleep-wake cycles.

Sleep deprivation offers other insights into consequences and benefits conferred.

Characteristics of sleep stages

NREM:

- 50% in Neonates
- 20% in Toddlers/young children
- 70-80% in Young adults
- Variable in Older adults

REM

- 50% in Neonates
- 20% in Young adults
- Variable in older adults
- Lasts approximately 10 minutes

Features of NREM stages:

Stage 1: takes approximate 1 to 7 minutes to commence. Light sleep, lack of awareness, easily roused

Stage 2: increasingly lack of sensitivity, harder to arouse from this state

Stage 3: After 20 minutes approximately, moderately deep sleep and person is hard to awaken. Breathing ad temperature decline

Stage 4: Deep sleep. Very difficult to awaken. Sleep walking, talking, nightmares may occur in this stage.

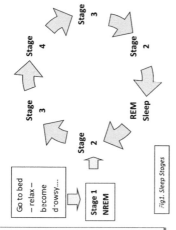

Go to bed – relax – become drowsy….

Stage 1 NREM

Stage 2

Stage 3

Stage 4

Stage 3

Stage 2

REM Sleep

Fig1. Sleep Stages

Stages of sleep

Non rapid eye movement (NREM) sleep:

Occurs first and has four stages moving from each sequentially i.e. 1 to 2 to 3 etc. Termed 'orthodox' sleep.

- One cycle of NREM leads to REM sleep stage.
- NREM stages 1 to 4 lasts approximately 40 minutes. In total whole cycle lasts approximately 90 minutes. (*NB some books combine stages 3 and 4*).
- Cycles repeated four or five times in a night period.
- Time in stages 3 and 4 decline as the night progresses.
- Progressive muscle relaxation and tension.
- Blood pressure, heart rate and respiratory rate decrease.
- Hormones released: Gonadotrophic hormones (linked to sex hormones) and growth hormone.

Rapid eye movement (REM) sleep:

Known as paradoxical sleep as the brain pattern resembles the awake state. Paradoxically a person in REM sleep is hard to arouse.

- Oxygen consumption is high.
- Increase in blood pressure and heart and respiratory rates (Fig. 1).
- Facial twitches but loss of skeletal muscle tone.
- Dreaming occurs in this stage.

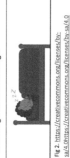

FIGURE 6.2 Physiology of sleep

Surgical patients

Often effected by disrupted sleep due to:

- Hospital factors (inpatient)
- Pain
- Restricted positioning
- Possible hypoxia or hypercapnia
- Medications (eg. opioids which induce drowsiness)
- Post-operative monitoring (vital signs)

See 'Ward Good Sleep Checklist' (Norton et al., 2015)

Consequences of fatigue and sleep deprivation:

- Decreased anabolism and tissue repair
- Decreased ability to participate in post-operative exercises or activities

Intensive care/unconscious patients

Despite status there exist flucuations in episodes of sleep and arousal states. Even though non responsive to stimuli.

Intensive care units (ICU) sleep was shown to be of a poor quality, owing to:

- artificial light,
- increased noise,
- a consequence of critical illness itself, and
- treatment interventions.

Sleep is fragmented, with

- frequent arousals,
- an increase in stage 2 NREM sleep, a reduction or absence of stage 3 NREM and REM sleep,
- circadian rhythms is also erratic in ICU affecting metabolism and therapies such as antibiotics and nutrition (Tiruvoipati et al., 2019).

In critically ill patients, inadequate sleep was shown to be associated with:

- mood changes including anxiety, depression, psychosis, and delirium
- a reduced pain threshold
- impaired immunity and overall mortality

Nonpharmacological interventions proposed:

- weaning mechanical ventilation modes, eye masks and/or earplugs, massage, foot baths, music interventions and aromatherapy

SLEEP SITUATIONS AND ENVIRONMENTS

People with dementia

A person with dementia may have altered sleep-wake cycles and problems with sleeping duration. They may get up during the night and become disorientated on waking. They may also get dressed or try to leave the house. One consequence then is daytime tiredness and napping.

Proposed approach:

- Increase daytime activities within ability range and normalize a daylight-awake habit.
- Limit alcohol or caffeine especially in evenings.
- Promote 'sleep routines' or sleep hygiene practices
- Milky drinks contain tryptophan which induces sleep.
- Ensure safety and possibly a clock nearby to prompt to time.

Figure 1 Baby sleeping position: Feet to foot. (The LullabyTrust.org.uk)

Babies and Young Children

The current guidance is for babies to sleep on their backs (supine) position (NHS, 2018). A rare but serious concern is Sudden Infant Death Syndrome (SIDS). The following guidance promote safe sleeping and minimizes this.

- Place baby on their back to sleep, in a cot in the same room as the parent for the first 6 months. Avoid exposure to smoke (before during and after birth) from parent or others.
- Parents ought not share a bed with baby if they have been drinking alcohol, taken drugs, or smoke.
- Not to sleep with baby on a sofa or armchair.
- Don't let baby get too hot or cold.
- Blankets ought to be tucked in no higher than their shoulders.
- Ensure "feet to foot" position, with baby's feet at the end of the cot or basket.

FIGURE 6.3 Sleep situations and environments

SLEEP *HYGIENE* OR PROMOTION

Improving sleep – considerations
Aim: Build a relaxing environment conducive to sleep.

- *Regularity*: getting up and going to bed times.
- *Bedroom*: reserved for sleeping, avoid working/other activities.
- *Develop pre-sleep routine*:
  o Children: milky drink, bath, night clothes, story/song.
  o Adults: own routines/habits. Changes which disrupt e.g. entering hospital. Re-establish routines if possible.
- *Address problems*: pain relief, position, comfort measures
- *Minimise troublesome factors*: noise, timing of fluid intake, excessive exercise, caffeine or other stimulants.
- *If practiced*: support spiritual or religious observances and any measure to support mental or emotional calm.
- *Environment*: light, ventilation, temperature (including bedclothes) as much as possible.
- *Electronics*: minimise use (tablets/mobile phones or computers) as blue light emitted blocks sleep readiness/neurotransmitters.
https://www.sleepfoundation.org/articles/how-blue-light-affects-kids-sleep

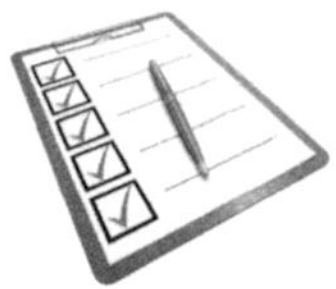

Copyright free: www.animatedheaven.weebly.com

Assessment of sleep: *What is normal?*

Holistic assessment to focus on what is usual versus unusual. Noting:

- Difficulty falling asleep
- Frequent waking during sleep cycle
- Early awakening
- Oversleeping
- Feel refreshed from sleep
- Dreams/nightmares
- Recent changes in sleep patterns
- Patterns known to affect their sleep (being alone)
- Diet/eating and exercise habits
- Worries or stresses/family/domestic/work problems
- Health (physical and mental) or physical impairments/limitations
- Regular or irregular medications (conventional or herbal/alternative including over the counter)

Sleep diary

- Ideally for one full week or more.
- Tool to determine main problems, impacts of interventions and progress. For children this needs to be age appropriate (drawings/ smiley faces etc.) or charts.

Advice to maintain this includes:

- Keep diary beside the bed
- Note activity and type of meal before bedtime
- Note time going to bed
- Note how long to fall asleep (when awake)
- If waking in the night – time what caused this
- Note how long and difficulty of getting back to sleep and any interventions undertaken
- Note time awoke next morning
- Note feeling of alertness and feeling rested or not and how long to get up
- Note total number of hours slept
- Note any dreams
- Note activities occurring during the day (work, meetings etc)
- Note feelings during the day (irritated, alert, relaxed or otherwise)
- Note any other useful aspects – arguments, menstruation, financial worries, medications taken

Published sleep assessment tools include:
Pittsburgh Sleep Quality Index. Epworth Sleepiness Scale. (BSSA, (ND). NHS Resource – Promoting Sleep: https://www.nhs.uk/oneyou/for-your-body/sleep-better/

FIGURE 6.4 Sleep hygiene or promotion

FACTORS DISRUPTING NORMAL SLEEP PATTERNS

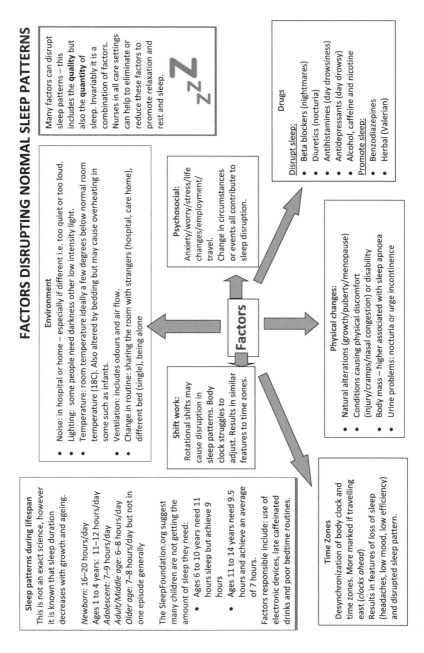

Sleep patterns during lifespan
This is not an exact science, however it is known that sleep duration decreases with growth and ageing.

Newborn: 16–20 hours/day
Ages 1 to 4 years: 11–12 hours/day
Adolescent: 7–9 hours/day
Adult/Middle age: 6–8 hours/day
Older age: 7–8 hours/day but not in one episode generally

The SleepFoundation.org suggest many children are not getting the amount of sleep they need:
- Ages 6 to 10 years need 11 hours sleep but achieve 9 hours
- Ages 11 to 14 years need 9.5 hours and achieve an average of 7 hours.

Factors responsible include: use of electronic devices, late caffeinated drinks and poor bedtime routines.

Time Zones
Desynchronization of body clock and time zones. More marked if travelling east (*clocks ahead*)
Results in features of loss of sleep (headaches, low mood, low efficiency) and disrupted sleep pattern.

Shift work:
Rotational shifts may cause disruption in sleep patterns. Body clock struggles to adjust. Results in similar features to time zones.

Factors

Environment
- Noise: in hospital or home – especially if different i.e. too quiet or too loud.
- Lighting: some people need darkness other low intensity light.
- Temperature: room temperature ideally a few degrees below normal room temperature (18C). Also altered by bedding but may cause overheating in some such as infants.
- Ventilation: includes odours and air flow.
- Change in routine: sharing the room with strangers (hospital, care home), different bed (single), being alone

Psychosocial:
Anxiety/worry/stress/life changes/employment/travel.
Change in circumstances or events all contribute to sleep disruption.

Physical changes:
- Natural alterations (growth/puberty/menopause)
- Conditions causing physical discomfort (injury/cramps/nasal congestion) or disability
- Body mass – higher associated with sleep apnoea
- Urine problems: nocturia or urge incontinence

Drugs
Disrupt sleep:
- Beta blockers (nightmares)
- Diuretics (nocturia)
- Antihistamines (day drowsiness)
- Antidepressants (day drowsy)
- Alcohol, caffeine and nicotine
Promote sleep:
- Benzodiazepines
- Herbal (Valerian)

Many factors can disrupt sleep patterns – this includes the **quality** but also the **quantity** of sleep. Invariably it is a combination of factors. Nurses in all care settings can help to eliminate or reduce these factors to promote relaxation and rest and sleep.

FIGURE 6.5 Factors disrupting normal sleep patterns

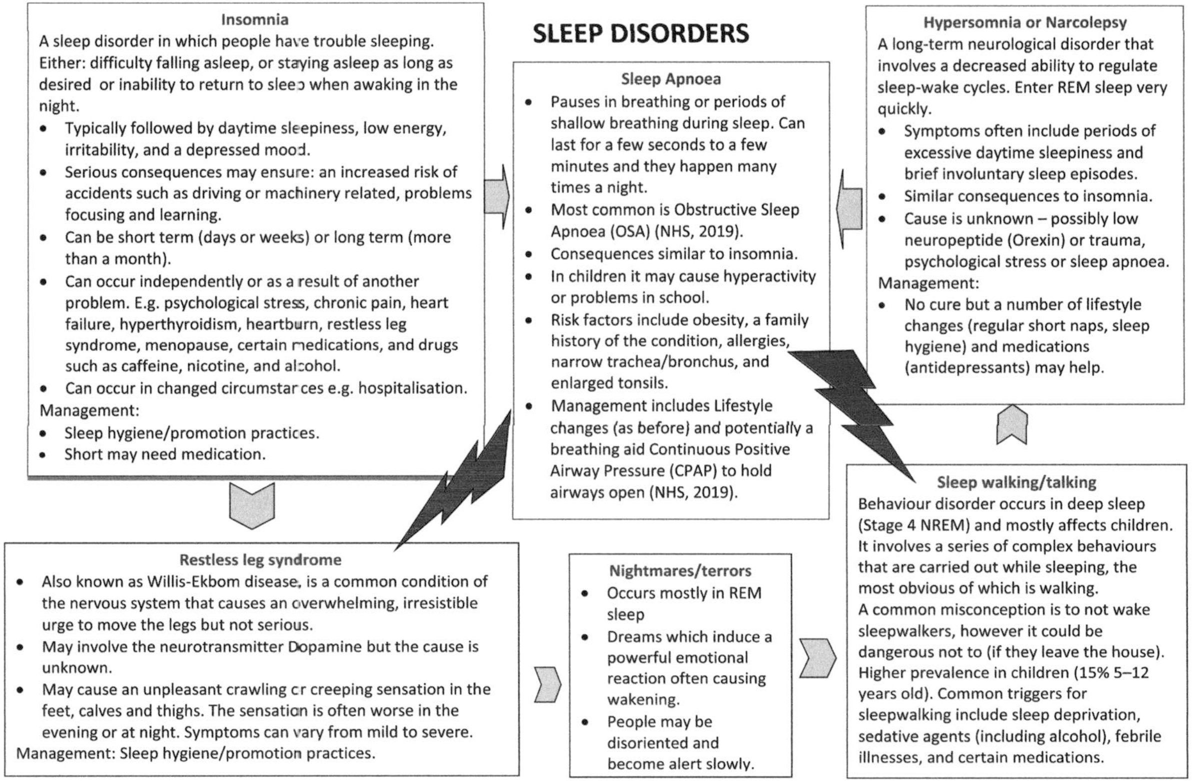

SLEEP DISORDERS

Insomnia

A sleep disorder in which people have trouble sleeping. Either: difficulty falling asleep, or staying asleep as long as desired or inability to return to sleep when awaking in the night.

- Typically followed by daytime sleepiness, low energy, irritability, and a depressed mood.
- Serious consequences may ensure: an increased risk of accidents such as driving or machinery related, problems focusing and learning.
- Can be short term (days or weeks) or long term (more than a month).
- Can occur independently or as a result of another problem. E.g. psychological stress, chronic pain, heart failure, hyperthyroidism, heartburn, restless leg syndrome, menopause, certain medications, and drugs such as caffeine, nicotine, and alcohol.
- Can occur in changed circumstances e.g. hospitalisation.

Management:
- Sleep hygiene/promotion practices.
- Short may need medication.

Sleep Apnoea

- Pauses in breathing or periods of shallow breathing during sleep. Can last for a few seconds to a few minutes and they happen many times a night.
- Most common is Obstructive Sleep Apnoea (OSA) (NHS, 2019).
- Consequences similar to insomnia.
- In children it may cause hyperactivity or problems in school.
- Risk factors include obesity, a family history of the condition, allergies, narrow trachea/bronchus, and enlarged tonsils.
- Management includes Lifestyle changes (as before) and potentially a breathing aid Continuous Positive Airway Pressure (CPAP) to hold airways open (NHS, 2019).

Hypersomnia or Narcolepsy

A long-term neurological disorder that involves a decreased ability to regulate sleep-wake cycles. Enter REM sleep very quickly.

- Symptoms often include periods of excessive daytime sleepiness and brief involuntary sleep episodes.
- Similar consequences to insomnia.
- Cause is unknown – possibly low neuropeptide (Orexin) or trauma, psychological stress or sleep apnoea.

Management:
- No cure but a number of lifestyle changes (regular short naps, sleep hygiene) and medications (antidepressants) may help.

Restless leg syndrome

- Also known as Willis-Ekbom disease, is a common condition of the nervous system that causes an overwhelming, irresistible urge to move the legs but not serious.
- May involve the neurotransmitter Dopamine but the cause is unknown.
- May cause an unpleasant crawling or creeping sensation in the feet, calves and thighs. The sensation is often worse in the evening or at night. Symptoms can vary from mild to severe.

Management: Sleep hygiene/promotion practices.

Nightmares/terrors

- Occurs mostly in REM sleep
- Dreams which induce a powerful emotional reaction often causing wakening.
- People may be disoriented and become alert slowly.

Sleep walking/talking

Behaviour disorder occurs in deep sleep (Stage 4 NREM) and mostly affects children. It involves a series of complex behaviours that are carried out while sleeping, the most obvious of which is walking.

A common misconception is to not wake sleepwalkers, however it could be dangerous not to (if they leave the house). Higher prevalence in children (15% 5–12 years old). Common triggers for sleepwalking include sleep deprivation, sedative agents (including alcohol), febrile illnesses, and certain medications.

FIGURE 6.6 Sleep disorders

Activity: now test yourself

1. Sleep is characterised by cycles of NREM and REM. Which of the following in relation to these cycles is true?

    a. REM and REM are equal in duration and depth and occur continuously throughout the night (ten minutes each).

    b. There are five cycles of REM to each one cycle of NREM.

    c. The whole cycle of NREM and REM takes approximately 90 minutes with four stages of NREM and one stage of REM.

    d. REM is responsible for nocturnally waking to urinate which occurs every three hours.

2. Identify four elements of a constructive pre-sleep routine to promote sleep in either children or adults.

3. During sleep apnoea the person:

    a. falls asleep without warning

    b. stops breathing for short periods during sleep

    c. gets up and starts walking about whilst sleeping

    d. talks incessantly in their sleep occasionally holding their breath before launching into a continual dialogue.

4. Milk is a drink often given to young children or adults as part of a bedtime routine. Why and what role does this have on sleep?

5. For patients in hospital, care homes or non-home environments sleep may be disrupted. Identify three key issues which may impact on the quality or quantity of sleep.

6. Which of the following is correct?

    a. Biorhythms are the same as circadian rhythms and seasonal rhythms.

    b. Biorhythms refer to the cyclic changes of peaks and troughs of energy and hormones levels within a person's body.

    c. Biorhythms can be interrupted by habits such as shift work or change in time zones.

    d. Biorhythms are connected to wakefulness and sleep and may be affected seasonally.

    e. All of the above.

    f. None of the above.

Answers

1. c).

   NREM means non rapid eye movement; these are incremental stages going into deeper sleep (stage 1 to 4 or conventional sleep), then back to stage 3 and 2 to REM (or rapid eye movements – paradoxical sleep).

2. Four elements of a constructive pre-sleep routine to promote sleep in either children or adults are:

   a) *regular routine most evenings*

   b) *relaxing environment*

   c) *bath*

   d) *reading or changing into night clothes.*

   There are many others: the aim is to create a relaxing atmosphere conducive to sleep.

3. b).

   'Apnoea' means cessation of breathing – this occurs for short periods and can be alarming for anyone listening to the sleeping person. If it is severe and disrupts sleep then assistance can be given to aid breathing (CPAP).

4. Milk is a long-known remedy for inducing sleepiness. It contains tryptophan, a dietary amino acid which is a component in serotonin, the neurotransmitter involved in sleep and part of the sleep–wake cycle.

5. Examples include:

   - *noise – environmental or from other people, or alternatively lack of noise if the home environment is near a busy urban area*

   - *light – which can impair relaxation and be a stimulus to the superchiasmatic nucleus (SCN) and induce wakefulness neurotransmitters*

- *disturbances – from staff or other people in the same environment, such as coughing, moving, going to the toilet*

- *temperature – too hot or too cold may impair sleep; this includes bedclothes as well as the environment.*

6. e).

They are all correct (apart from the 'none of the above'). There are a number of rhythms: female oestrogen cycles, seasonal cycles (linked to so-called seasonal affective disorder), circadian rhythms or diurnal rhythms... Biorhythms are a cyclic pattern which is important and they can be disrupted by aspects such as changes in time zones, shift work, or seasons.

Reflection: ask yourself

1. What do I know now that I didn't know before?

2. What am I confused/unclear about?

3. What areas do I need to focus on?

4. My action plan for further learning (make objectives SMART – Specific/Measurable/Achievable/Realistic/Time-bound):

Bibliography

Baker, F. C., de Zambotti, M., Colrain, I. M., and Bei, B. (2018) Sleep Problems during the Menopausal Transition: Prevalence, Impact, and Management Challenges. *Nature and Science of Sleep*, 10, 73–95. doi: 10.2147/NSS.S125807.

Bartel, K., and Gradisar, M. (2017) New Directions in the Link between Technology Use and Sleep in Young People. In: Nevšímalová, S., and Bruni, O. (eds.), *Sleep Disorders in Children*. Cham: Springer. doi: 10.1007/978-3-319-28640-2_4.

Béphage, G. (2005) Promoting Quality Sleep in Older People: The Nursing Care Role. *British Journal of Nursing*, 14(4), 205–210.

Bernhofer, E., Higgins, P., Daly, B., Burant, C., Hornick, T. (2014). Hospital lighting and its association with sleep, mood and pain in medical inpatients. *Journal of Advanced Nursing* 70(5): 1164–1173.

Blume, C., Del Giudice, R., Wislowska, M., Lechinger, J., and Schabus, M. (2015) Across the Consciousness Continuum – From Unresponsive Wakefulness to Sleep. *Frontiers in Human Neuroscience*, 9(105–110).

British Snoring and Sleep Apnoea Association (BSSA) (n.d.) What is Sleep Apnoea. [online]: https://britishsnoring.co.uk/snoring_&_sleep _apnoea/what_is_sleep_apnoea.php. Accessed 02.04.20.

Bruneau, E. G., Pluta, A., and Saxe, R. (2012) Distinct Roles of the 'Shared Pain' and 'Theory of Mind' Networks in Processing Others' Emotional Suffering. *Neuropsychologia*, 50(2), 219–231. doi: 10.1016/j. neuropsychologia.2011.11.008.

Diabetes UK. Hyperglycaemia (Hypers). https://www.diabetes.org.uk/gu ide-to-diabetes/complications/hypers. (2020) Accessed 23.08.20.

Gordon, A. L., and Gladman, J. R. (2010) Sleep in Care Homes. *Reviews in Clinical Gerontology*, Cambridge University Press, 20(4), 309–316.

Guyton, A. C., and Hall, J. E. (2020) *Textbook of Medical Physiology*, 14th edn. Philadelphia: Elsevier.

Guzmán-Vélez, E., Feinstein, J. S., and Tranel, D. (2014) Feelings without Memory in Alzheimer Disease. *Cognitive and Behavavioural Neurology*, 27(3), 117–29. doi: 10.1097/WNN.0000000000000020.

International Association for the Study of Pain (IASP) (2019) IASP's Proposed New Definition of Pain Released for Comment. [online]: https://www.iasp-pain.org/PublicationsNews/NewsDetail.aspx?I temNumber=9218. Accessed 28.04.20.

Lavoie, C. J., Zeidler, M. R., and Martin, J. L. (2018) Sleep and Aging. *Sleep Science Practice*, 2, 3. doi: 10.1186/s41606-018-0021-3.

Marieb, E. (2018) *Human Anatomy and Physiology*, 11th edn. London: Pearson.

National Health Service. (2017) Health Survey for England (HSE). [online]: https://digital.nhs.uk/pubs/hse2017. Accessed 28.04.20.

National Health Service (2018) Reduce the Risk of Sudden Infant Death Syndrome (SIDS). [online]: https://www.nhs.uk/conditions/pregnancy-and-baby/reducing-risk-cot-death/. Accessed 02/04/20.

National Health Service (2019) Sleep Apnoea. [online]: https://www.nhs.uk/conditions/sleep-apnoea/. Accessed 02.04.20.

National Institute for Health and Care Excellence (NICE) (2007) *Acutely Ill Patients in Hospital: Recognition of and Response to Acute Illness in Adults in Hospital*. London: NICE.

National Institute for Health and Care Excellence (NICE) (2012). *Meningitis (bacterial) and meningococcal septicaemia in children and young people*. https://www.nice.org.uk/guidance/qs19/chapter/quality-statement-5-lumbar-puncture-for-suspected-bacterial-meningitis. Accessed 22.06.20.

National Institute for Health and Care Excellence (NICE) (2015). *Pressure ulcers*. https://www.nice.org.uk/guidance/qs89/chapter/Quality-statement-8-Pressure-redistribution-devices. Accessed 27.07.20.

National Institute for Health and Care Excellence (NICE) (2020a) *Acutely Ill Adult in Hospital Overview*. London. [online]: file:///C:/Users/tina2/AppData/Local/Temp/acutely-ill-patients-in-hospital-acutely-ill-patients-in-hospital-overview-1.pdf. Accessed 22.06.2020.

National Institute for Health and Care Excellence (NICE) (2020b) Hypoglycaemia. https://bnf.nice.org.uk/treatment-summary/hypoglycaemia.html. Accessed 22.06.2020.

Norton, C., Flood, D., Brittin, A., and Miles, J. (2015) Improving Sleep for Patients in Acute Hospitals. *Nursing Standard*, 29(28), 35–42. doi: 10.7748/ns.29.28.35.e8947

Nursing and Midwifery Council (NMC) (2018) *Future Nurse Proficiencies*. London. [online]: https://www.nmc.org.uk/globalassets/sitedocuments/education-standards/future-nurse-proficiencies.pdf. Accessed 03.07.20.

Patel, M., Chipman, J., Carlin, B. W., and Shady, D. (2008) Sleep in the Intensive Care Unit. *Critical Care Nursing*, 31(4), 309–318.

Pilkington, S. (2013) Causes and Consequences of Sleep Deprivation in Hospitalised Patients. *Nursing Standard*, 27(49), 35–42. doi: 10.7748/ns2013.08.27.49.35.e7649.

Pisani, M. A., Friese, R. S., Gehlbach, B. K., Schwab, R. J., Weinhouse, G. L., and Jones, S. F. (2015) Sleep in the Intensive Care Unit. *American Journal of Respiratory & Critical Care Medicine*, 191(7), 731–738. doi: 10.1164/rccm.201411-2099CI.

Price, C., Hoggart, B., Olukoga, O., de Williams, A., Bottle, A. (2012) *National Pain Audit 2010–2012*. London: The British Pain Society.

Resuscitation Council (UK) (2015) Resuscitation Guidelines. [online]: https://www.resus.org.uk/library/2015-resuscitation-guidelines. Accessed 27.06.20.

Royal College of Nursing (2015) Pain Knowledge and Skills Framework for the Nursing Team. [online]: https://www.britishpainsociety.org/static/uploads/resources/files/RCN_KSF_2015.pdf. Accessed 20.05.20.

Slate, M. (2019) Neurotransmitters: Their Role in the Body. RN.org. [online]: https://www.rn.org/courses/coursematerial-150.pdf. Accessed 15.04.20.

The Lullaby Trust (2019) The Best Sleeping Position for Your Baby. [online]: https://www.lullabytrust.org.uk/safer-sleep-advice/sleeping-position/. Accessed 24.04.20.

Tiruvoipati, R., Mulder, J., and Haji, K. (2019) Improving Sleep in Intensive Care Unit: An Overview of Diagnostic and Therapeutic Options. *Journal of Patient Experience*, 1–6. [online]: https://journals.sagepub.com/doi/pdf/10.1177/2374373519882234. Accessed 26.04.20.

Tortora, G., and Derrickson. G. (2019) *Introduction to the Human Body*, 11th edn. New York: Wiley.

Index

Page numbers in *italics* denote figures.

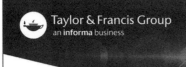